100 practical tips for a Highly Sensitive Persons' home in 20 days
by Alain de Raymond

I0440611

To everyone who supported me while writing this book – especially my parents.

Table of Contents

Introduction: the HSP home in 100 tips

Living as a very/highly sensitive person (HSP) is difficult to imagine for persons who are not as sensitive as HSPs. The noise a bird makes while everyone is talking. The need to retreat after a long meeting. Feeling anti-social but loving deep conversations. **Living is different**.

A key point for HSPs is to feel good in your own house. It's your retreat. It's where you live. It's where you spend most of your time. If you can't find **a good balance** for yourself in your own home, then where will you find refuge?

Many books were written about sensitivity. However, most tend to cover relationships as well as self-acceptance tips. The purpose of this book is to give **practical tips** you may not have thought of. Tips making your life as an HSP a little easier. And all those 'littles' combined, will give you a 'big' extra life quality back.

HSPs have a lot in common, but **each HSP is different**. Some are introverted, others extraverted. Some write books, other can't drive a car and HSP children deserve a special approach. Select and apply the tips that work out well for you.

So let's see **100 tips** for your home. We start with what you can do now. We'll continue with tips for later in the day, and then with tips for the coming days, weeks and months, with a focus on the first 20 days. Also check the useful links in the bonus sections, as well as other practical tips for choosing a home and how to live with children.

Here are two links to help you before we start:

-Here's a **20% discount** on my 1.5 hour course how to deal with your sensitivity. At work, dating, travelling, and many more subjects.

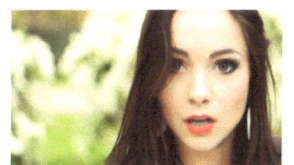

udemy.com/highly-sensitive-persons-how-to-deal-with-your-sensitivity/?couponCode=BOOK-CODE23

-If Adam Smith is the father of the free markets theories, then **Dr Elaine Aron** is the mother of the study on Highly Sensitive Persons. Do the HSP test and find many other tips on **her website**.

hsperson.com

So let's get started!

Alain

1. Right now

So let's start with what you can do right now, while you're reading this book. So what can you do in this moment to improve your HSP life?

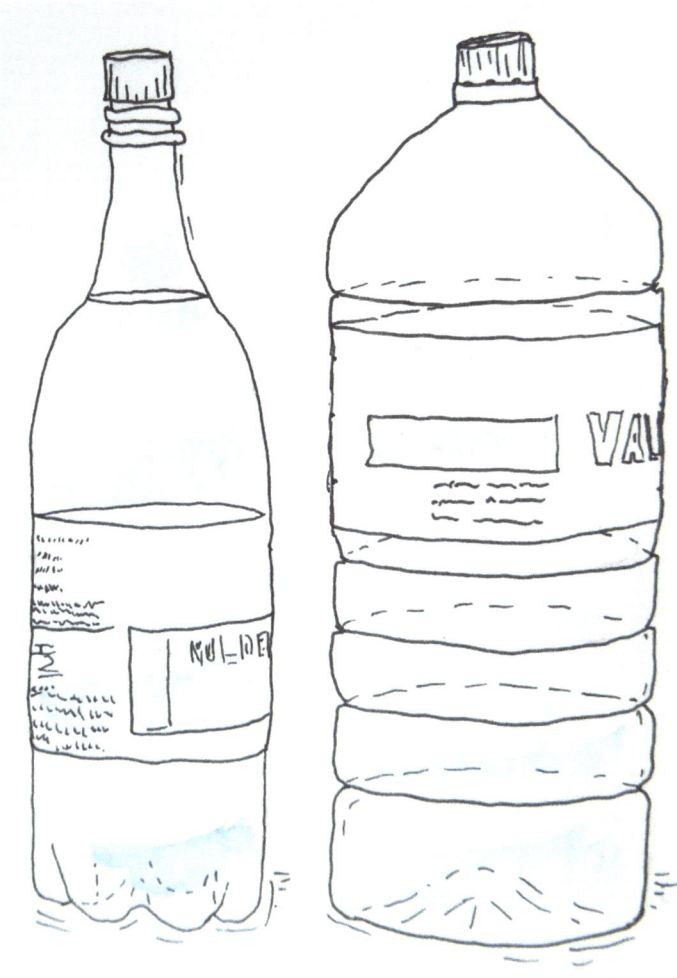

Tip 1: Grab a bottle of **water** and **drink**. Water is one of the best drinks there is. Later on, check out how much you should drink according to your height and weight. Or ask your family doctor. Water also has positive psychological effects, according to some therapists.

Tip 2: Listening to **music** while reading this book? Great, music can have a calming effect. So make some mood playlists, depending on which emotion you're feeling. Make sure to have your '**after-work-playlist**' ready for your next working day.

Tip 3: Another good idea is to have **white noise** ready. Test the different types, for example raindrops, piano music or flute music. The white noise is louder than those small sounds you might hear in your home. Natural noise is even better. Like the waves of the sea. Also, don't hesitate to ask others to turn their volume down. Or put your headphones on.

Tip 4: What's the temperature in the room? And in the other rooms? HSPs are sensitive to temperature changes. So make sure the **temperature** is **consistent** in the rooms you're spending the most time. So set it right. And make sure you wear the appropriate clothes according to the weather.

Tip 5: How is the room you're in? Tidy? If not, make sure to **tidy up**. HSPs notice objects lying in the wrong place, called visual clutter. Which will make you more tired. So put your clothes lying around in the closet, where they belong.

However, don't exaggerate. A home can't always be perfectly tidy. Especially if you have children. Teach them to tidy up after themselves. A 'tidy-up-song' may help.

2. Later today

Now that you've tidied up the room, and maybe some other rooms, and taken a rest, it's time to continue our tour to make your home HSP-friendlier. Let's start with an unexpected room…

Tip 6: Where do you go when you're overwhelmed? HSPs are easily overwhelmed. So one fo the best places to shelter is… the **bathroom**. Whenever you're overwhelmed, even if it's at someone else's place, is the bathroom. No one will ask questions. And you can stay there as long as you want - to recover.

Tip 7: Is your phone near? Is the **ringtone** nice? Well, if not, grab it and change it into something nice. Not a sudden one. Or just put it on vibration only, so you won't have to switch it off. It's already scary enough to be called at any moment of the day.

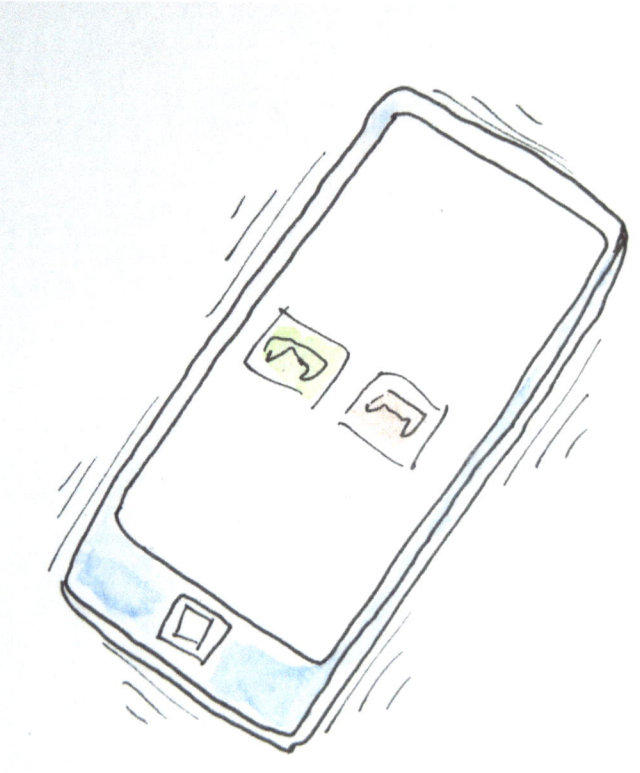

Tip 8: Do you have a fixed phone? Place it in a quiet place in your home. It can be difficult for HSPs to focus on the voice of the caller if there are many surrounding sounds. So **pick up** in a **quiet** spot, and wait a bit before picking up so you can switch your mind to the phone call.

Tip 9: And if someone else is calling, make sure to put some **distance** between you and the **caller**. It can be very annoying to be obliged to listen to only one part of the conversation. Also, when someone is texting or playing a game and there's a bleep for every tick, it can tick you off. So take a distance - it is your right.

Tip 10: Let's check your computer before we go eating. And your smartphone - if you have one. Electronic equipment usually gives lots of stimuli, like sounds or smells. Which is something HSPs should try to **limit**. So less time on your **computer** and your **smartphone** is good.

Tip 11: Of course, it's easier said than done. But the internet can help you. For example, with **social media**. There are many applications to limit the time you're looking at funny movies, political opinions and your friends' meals. For example, use apps like SelfControl (selfcontrolapp.com) or Cold Turkey (getcoldturkey.com).

Tip 12: And **disconnect** as much as possible. Or just don't connect. Take some time to de-friend, to unlike, and to leave the groups on your social media from time to time. Same goes for email **subscriptions**. If you didn't read the 10 previous newsletters, you won't read the next one.

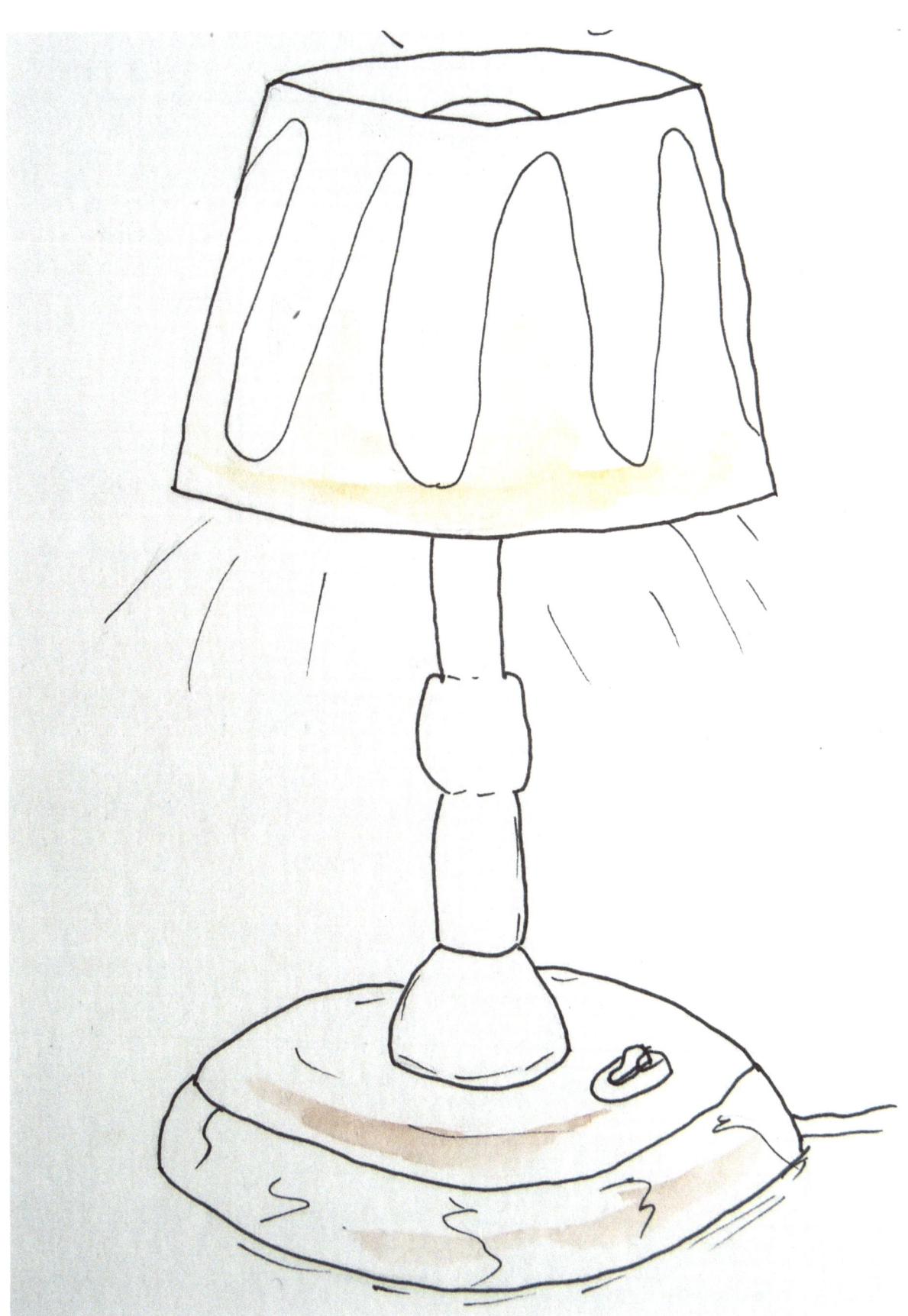

Tip 13: While you're disconnecting, **type slower**. HSPs tend to be perfectionists. And so some try to type as fast as possible. That's the opposite of what you should do. Typing slower will relax you.

Tip 14: Is it already dark when you're reading this book? Well, your smartphone and your computer don't know that, even though they have a built-in clock. Their screens don't adapt to the time of the way. Meaning your eyes will get tired very quickly when it gets dark. Luckily, there's an application for that: download and install f.lux (justgetflux.com). It will **dim the light** at the end of the day.

Tip 15: Dimming the light isn't the only thing apps can do for you. Do you sometimes get upset by the **flashy internet advertisements**? Usually, they're loud, have bright lights and disrupt your routine. Everything an HSP would want to avoid. And there's an app for that as well: AdBlock (getadblock.com).

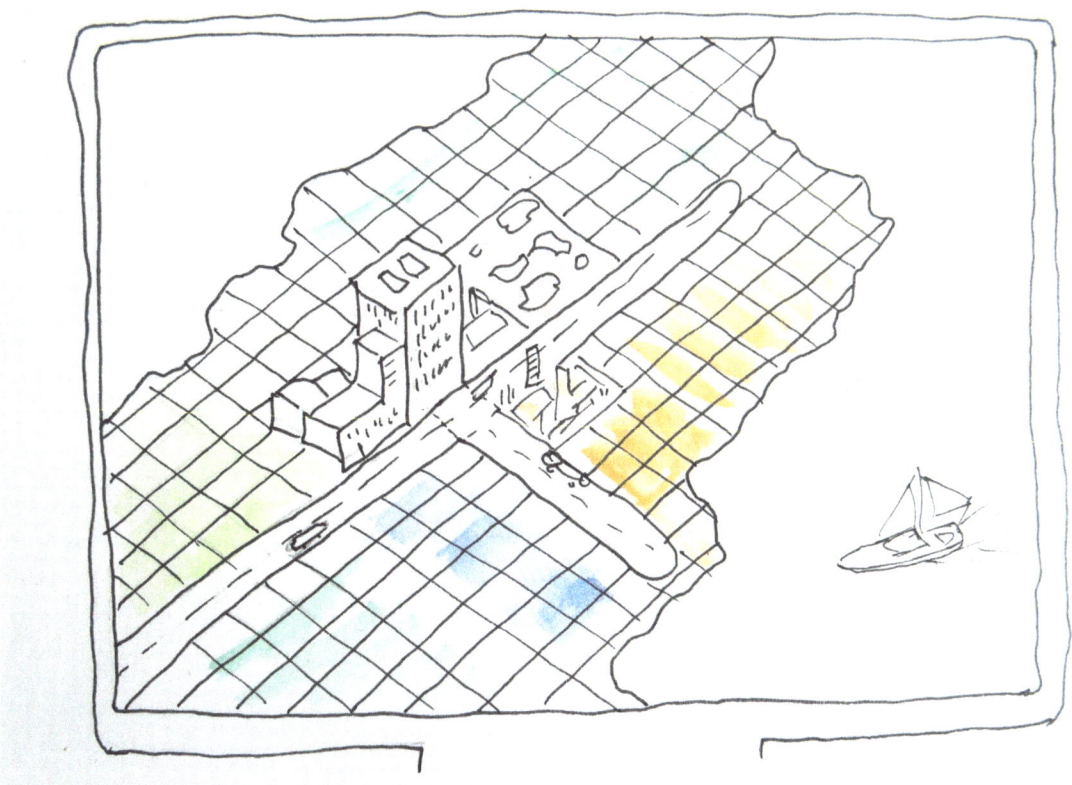

Tip 16: Do you play **games** sometimes? Select the ones that are HSP-friendly. Don't shoot zombies. But rather games that allow you to build cities or other strategic games.

Let's see how you can make your evening more HSP-friendly in the next chapter…

3. Tonight

Time to start preparing for your well-deserved dinner. And here's a first important tip.

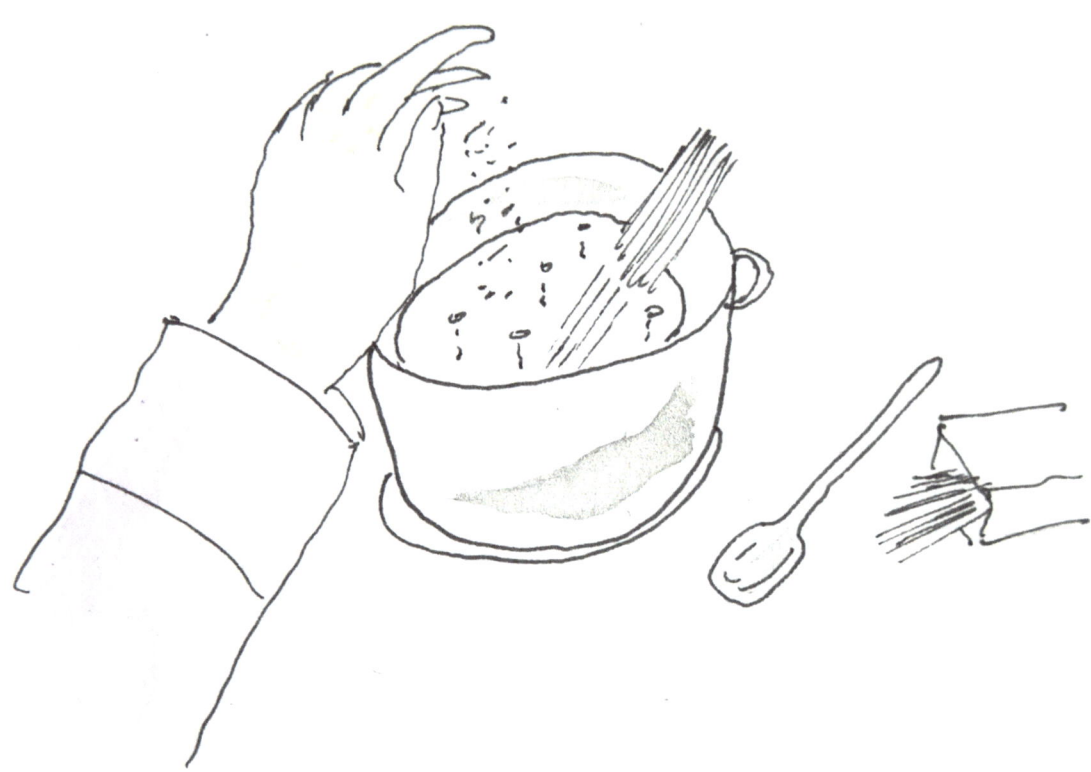

Tip 17: Who cooks at your place? Is it a member of your family? Or the local pizza provider? The best way to take care of yourself is to **cook yourself**. Or, at least, to get involved. You know your body best. Mind which ingredients or spices you're sensitive to. And if you're not cooking, make sure you inform the cook.

Tip 18: While you're cooking, know that many HSPs are **more sensitive to smells** than non-HSPs. This can be an advantage: you'll be the first one to notice if food burns. Or if something is rotten. Also use your nose to cook. If something doesn't smell nice, better not eat it.

Tip 19: Eating with others can be overwhelming. So **avoid extra noises** like the radio or the television playing.

Tip 20: Drinking your soup? Or eating ice cream? Pay attention to the **temperature** of what you're eating. If you know you get a headache after drinking something cold, just wait a little.

Tip 21: A good way to finish your meal is by **drinking tea**, even though you have to wait until it has a nice temperature. Herbal tea is a great idea. Avoid too strong or dark tea or too much sugar in the tea. Use honey instead of sugar to sweeten your tea. It's healthier.

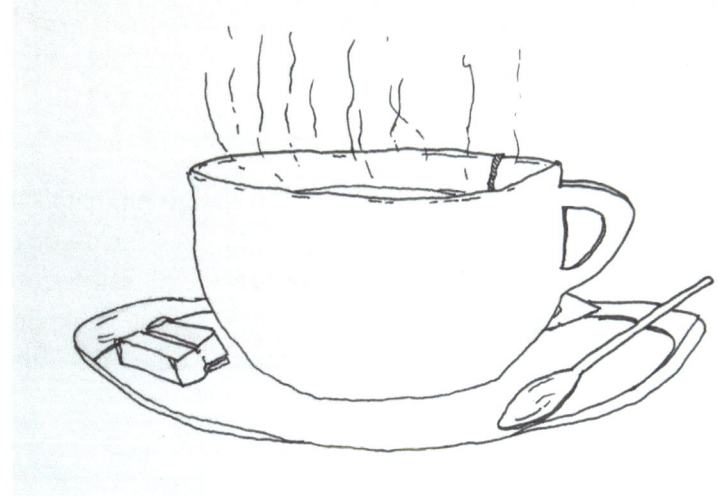

Tip 22: Some persons have the habit of watching the news just after eating. It's good to be informed, right? For HSPs, it's important to **select the news**. Don't watch or read popular news stories. Bad news sells. And it makes people want to know what they should be afraid of the day after.

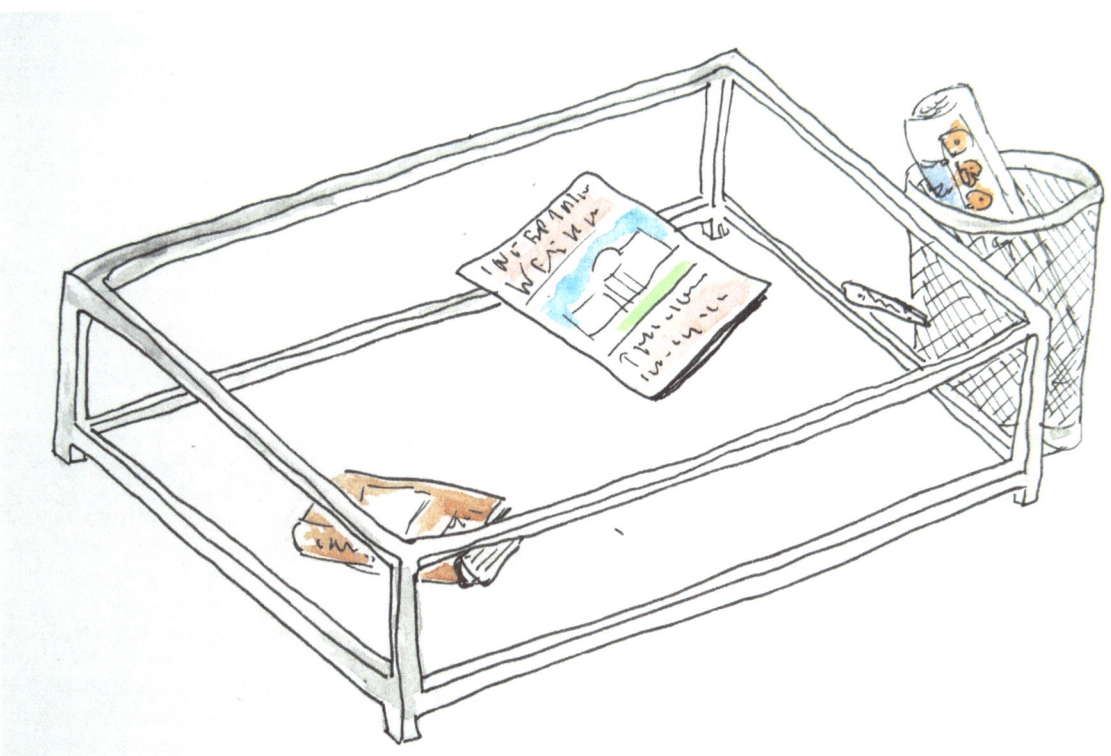

HSPs are particularly **vulnerable to bad news**. Because in prehistoric times, their task was to spot danger. Like wild animals or other tribes. Also, HSPs are more empathic. So no need to feel empathy for persons you don't know in the latest new drama. Even though it sounds hard, it's their problem and not yours.

Tip 23: Not exposing yourself to bad news doesn't mean you can't get informed. Non-daily serious magazines, in-depth documentaries and psychology or feel-good magazines are excellent options. Rule of thumb is: the more it's commercial and popular, the worse it is for HSPs. So tabloids are a no-go, but **serious newspapers** might still be good.

Tip 24: So maybe, instead of watching the news, you want to see a good **movie** on TV? Well, avoid horror movies, thrillers and violence. You'll get a lot of needless stimuli and you'll feel empathy for people you don't know. If you're hooked on a zombie series, watch them before the evening starts. You'll probably sleep better.

Tip 25: Talking about **television**: don't switch it on just to find something to watch. Or just to have something in the background going. Check the guide online or in the newspaper before switching it on. No need to get irritated by the pointless commercial shows, word-filled talkshows, the channels' different volumes, and the annoying and disrupting advertisements. If you want background noise, check the tips in the first chapter.

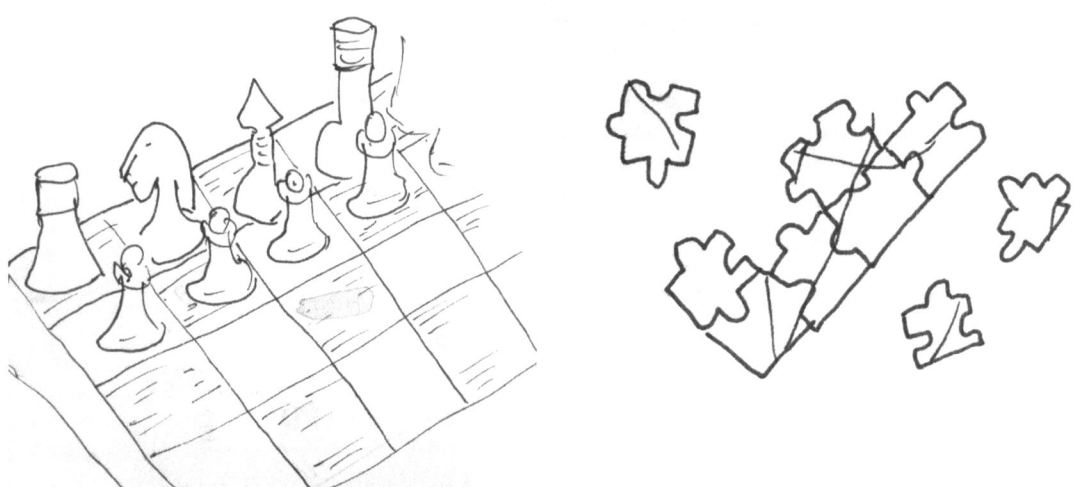

Tip 26: So what can you do instead of watching television? **Games** are a great thing to do. Try those you can play on your own. Like a puzzle, it's nice to see the result at the end. If you're playing with others, choose strategy games like chess. But choose a patient partner. You don't want to be pushed.

If you're more than three, **splitting up** is a good idea. Lots of people putting you under pressure to make quick decisions can lead to overwhelming situations for HSPs. Which is certainly not a good idea in the evening.

Tip 27: One last tip before we get ready for bed: switch off your **overhead lamps**. They're very intense and many HSPs dislike them. They flicker or make annoying noises. At work, try to find a spot near natural light and bring a desk lamp if you need to.

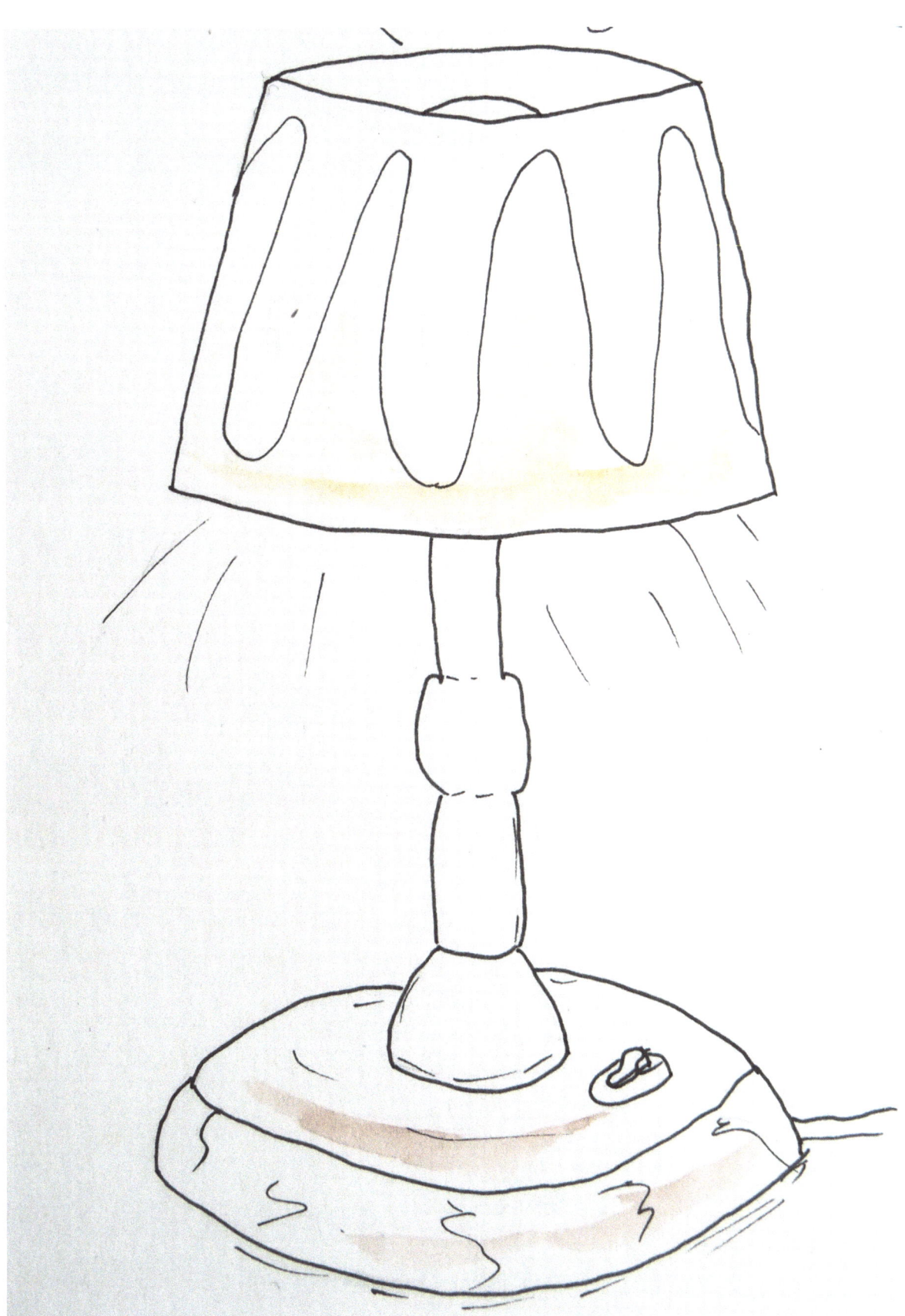

4. Bedtime

Let's prepare to go to bed. As an HSP, one does not simply go to bed. You can improve your sleep with the following tips.

Tip 28: Get into your **pre-bed routine** an hour or two before you enter your bed. Avoid getting too many stimuli in. So no difficult games or death metal music just before sleeping.

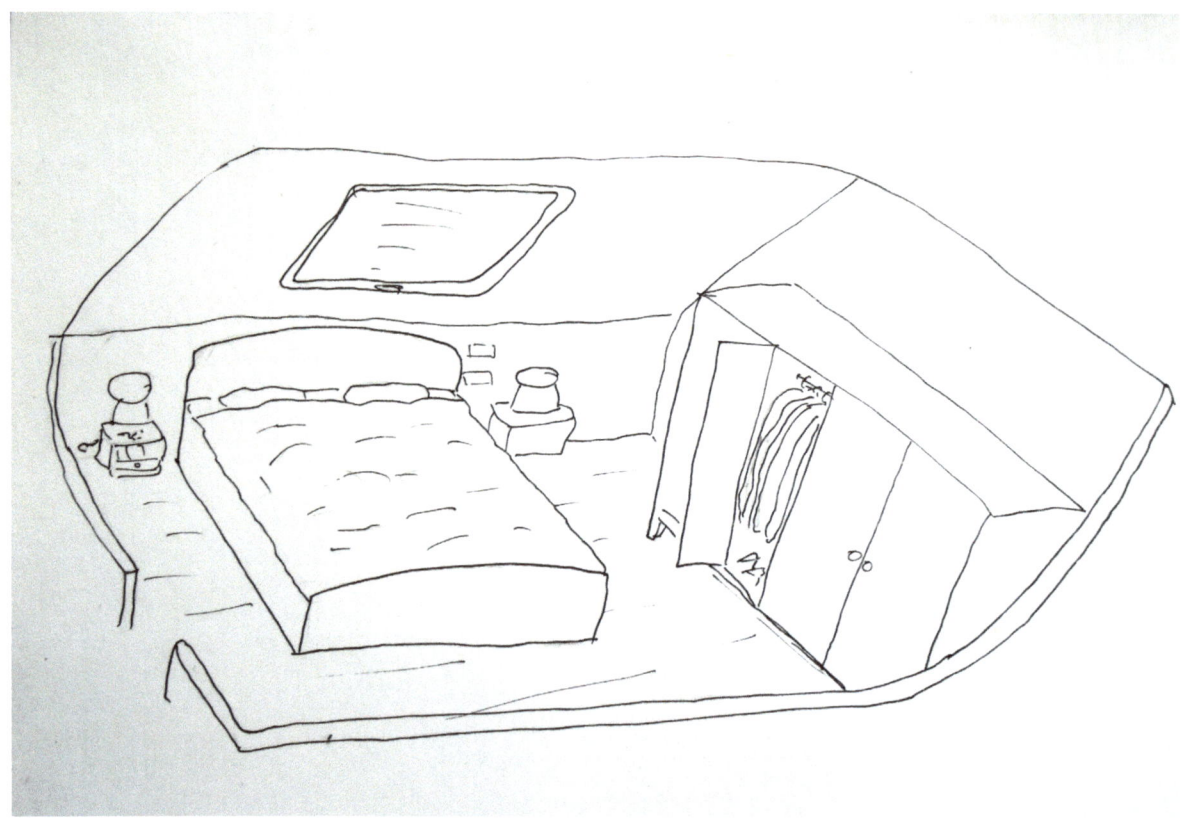

Tip 29: One way to start getting ready for bed is by **bathing or showering**. It's a way to show respect to your body, and to reconnect if you forced it. Make it last as much as it needs to last. The sound of your shower can relax you.

Tip 30: Another option is to **write a journal**. It also has a calming effect. It connects your thoughts and your body. Thoughts circulating in your head through the day will find rest in your journal.

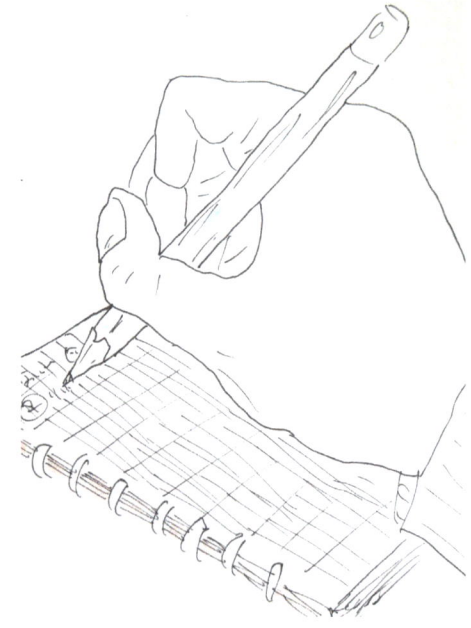

Tip 31: What you can also do, is to give or receive **massages**. You can focus on your or your partner's body, which is very relaxing. Giving yourself a massage is an alternative. Don't hesitate to have massages also during the day, or to take a massage class in your neighbourhood.

Tip 32: **Sleep in a bed**. Don't sleep in a couch. They're not made for sleeping. Also check if your mattress is comfortable to you.

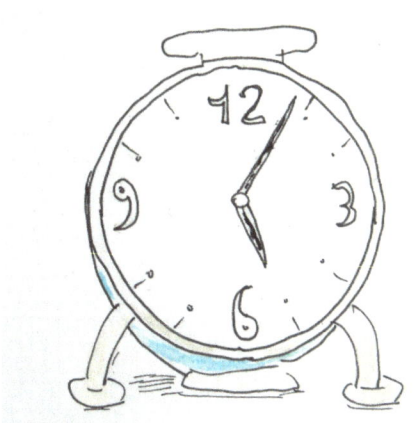

Tip 33: Just before you start sleeping, check your **alarm clock**. Is it a noisy one? Trade it for an alarm that has a nice sound. Alarms have a disrupting effect. And an over-used snooze button.

Tip 34: Time to sleep. It's important to get **enough sleep**. HSPs need more sleep than non-HSPs to process all the stimuli they received. Short nights can result in bad temper, irritation and a lack of concentration. So when friends brag about how little sleep they got the night before, there's no need to imitate them.

Have a good night!

5. Tomorrow morning

Tip 35: Did you sleep well last night? Any dreams? HSPs can remember their **dreams** better than non-HSPs. And yes, sometimes, they're crazy. Give them a positive ending when you're awake, or write them down.

Tip 36: How is the light in the bedroom? **Natural light is good**. Even if you prefer the quiet nights, make sure to enjoy the natural light during the day. Not having enough daylight can weaken your immune system and make you more vulnerable to diseases like depression.

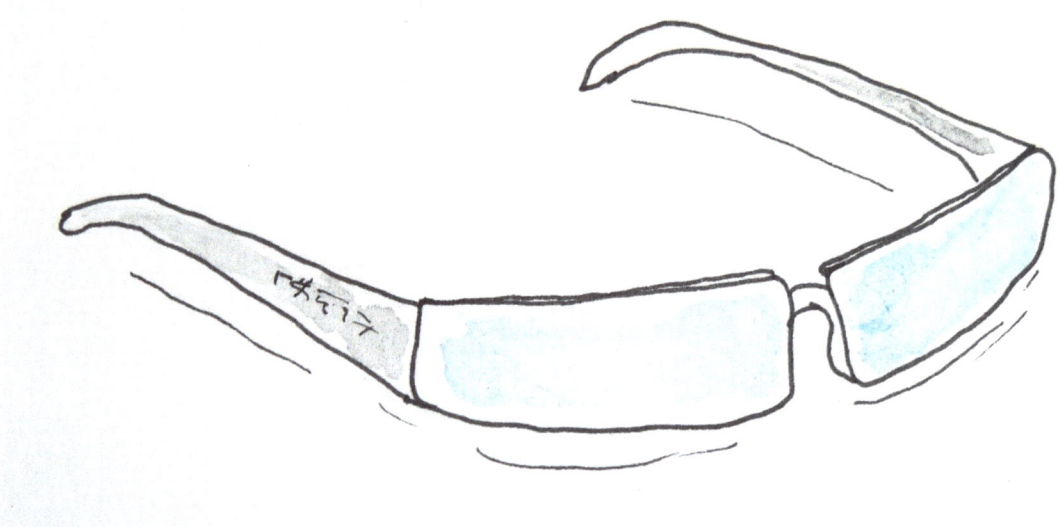

Tip 37: Mind this as well outside. If you can choose between a dark metro station or a 10-minute walk, you'll know what to do. If it's too bright in one of your rooms, make sure to put **sunglasses** within your grasp. Outside, don't forget to carry a hat with your sunglasses.

Tip 38: Once you've written your dreams and gotten comfortable with the light, it's time to do your **wake-up routine**. Waking up 10-20 minutes earlier will avoid you to rush into work or other activities. A good morning routine is to tidy up a room.

Tip 39: Just before getting off to work, make sure to prepare a **food bag**. If the weather is nice, you can eat outside. Alternatively, you can eat in your car if you have one.

Also, bring **healthy snacks** for when you're getting hungry in the afternoon. Some HSPs can't concentrate anymore with an empty belly. It's called being 'hangry', hunger and angry together. So better avoid it. Let's go to work now!

6. Tomorrow evening

Once you're back from work, it's time to think on making your house HSP-friendly again. Since we've already seen what to do in the evening in a previous chapter, let's focus on one aspect: online shopping.

Tip 40: Buying products online has many advantages for HSPs. No need to go to big shops like Ikea full of people and no exits. Also, you can check reviews so you will have some help to choose between too many products. Choices aren't easy for HSPs. And you won't have to deal with pushy salespersons. So, **shop online**! Be careful which sites to use: Amazon might be a good start.

Tip 41: First thing to buy on the internet: a **wake-up light**. It's much more pleasant to wake up to a changing light than to a changing sound. Buy one that can be customised to your needs.

Tip 42: Second product: a **clock** that doesn't make noise. Unless it calms you. If you prefer to wake up to noise, make sure it includes an alarm that can be customised. Choose a nice tune to wake up to.

Tip 43: Third product: a nice **doorbell**. If you have a doorbell that makes a horrible, sudden noise, it's time to change. Nowadays these can also be customised. For example, your favourite song becoming slowly louder. Make sure you can distinguish the sound from the others in your home. Goodbye surprise feelings!

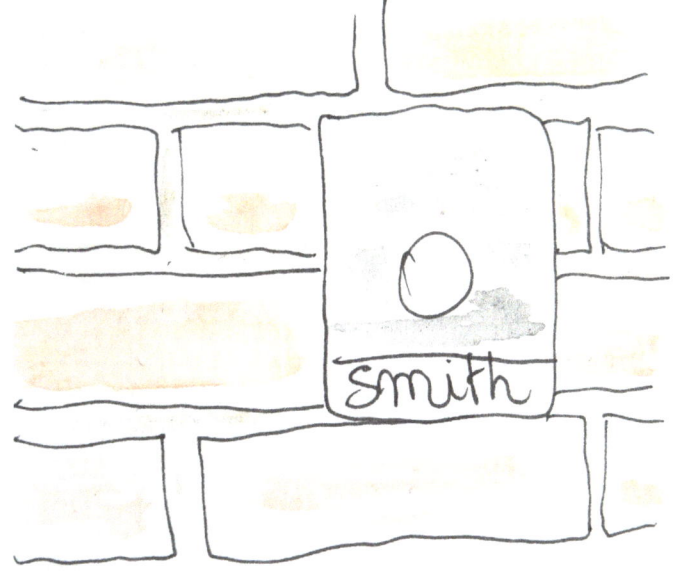

Tip 44: Fourth product: **menstruation cups**. Well, for women only - obviously. Menstruation cups are better than other chemical things. They're reusable, cheaper and last longer.

Tip 45: Fifth product: an **ashtray**. If you haven't already got one. Place it strategically on your terrace or on another spot outside. So if you have smoking guests, you can gently refer them to that spot. The intense smell of cigarettes gets many HSPs worked up. And of course, it's better not to smoke yourself.

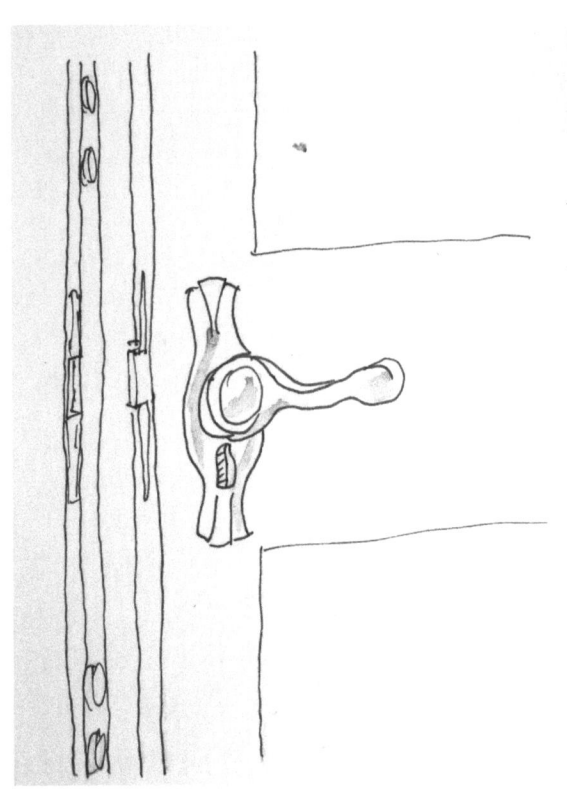

Tip 46: Last product to order: **anti-slam pads**. Annoyed by doors making wobbling noises all the time, with or without slamming? Either you can buy new doors or just install 'felt pads', little door cushions spread on the inside of the door. It's definitely cheaper.

Tip 47: An idea to thing about: how about all the products in your home you don't need? You can give them away to friends, but also sell them on second-hand sites like eBay. Like if you feel your **TV** doesn't add anything to your life, why not **sell** it?

7. Next weekend

Finally, the weekend has come. Some extra time to think about what you can change to your home. Think also about the tips you read about in this book. Which ones can you apply in a different way, so they work out well for you? Take enough time to reflect - HSPs usually love reflecting.

Let's get on with the tips. Let's go buy provisions for the week in your supermarket, and then see some practical tips for your hobbies.

Tip 48: But first, **make a list** of what you need. When you're in a supermarket, you might be overwhelmed so make sure you know all the things you need. Also, buy enough so you don't have to go too often.

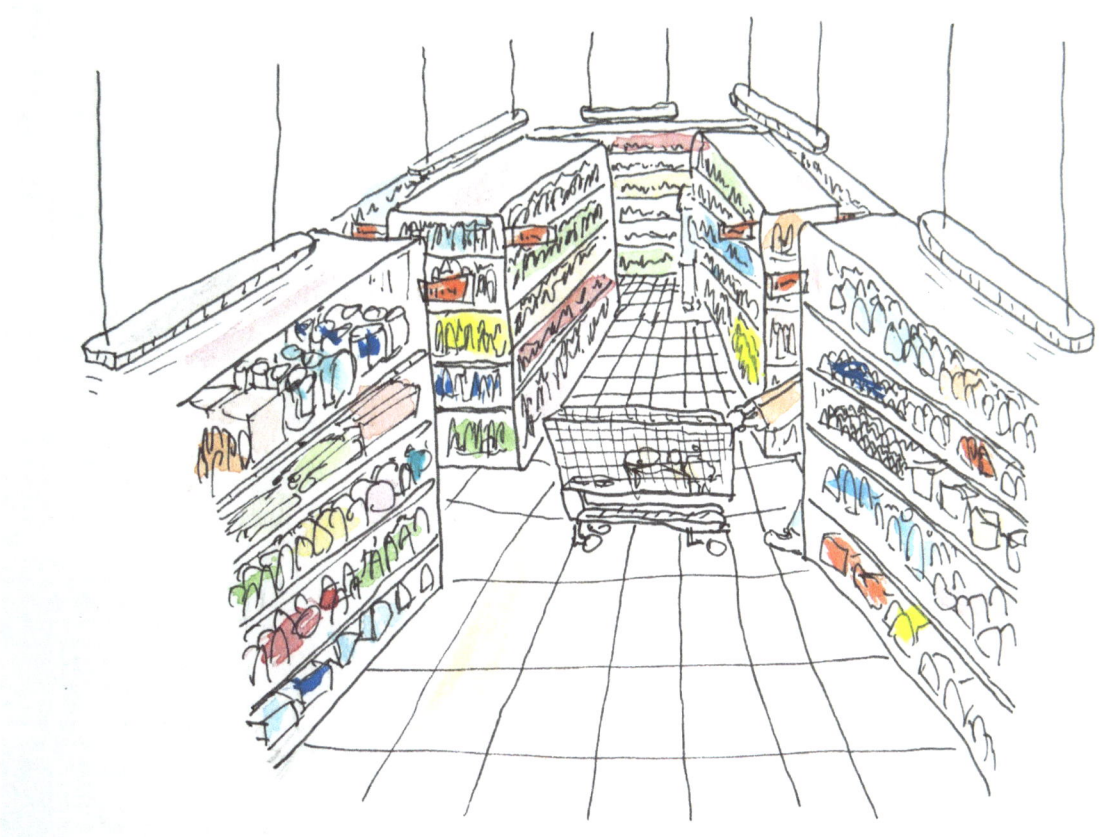

Tip 49: The **supermarket**. Artificial light. Bad acoustics. People going in all directions at the same time. Flashy products and their packages fighting all together for your attention. Noise everywhere - even the fridges make horrible noises. Better limit your time there.

Tip 50: If you decided to go, shop during the calm hours. In the early morning or around noon is usually calmer. Also consider going to smaller shops. Some supermarkets offer **online shopping**, so you'll only need to collect what you bought. Goodbye queues! Some even get your food delivered at home - check it.

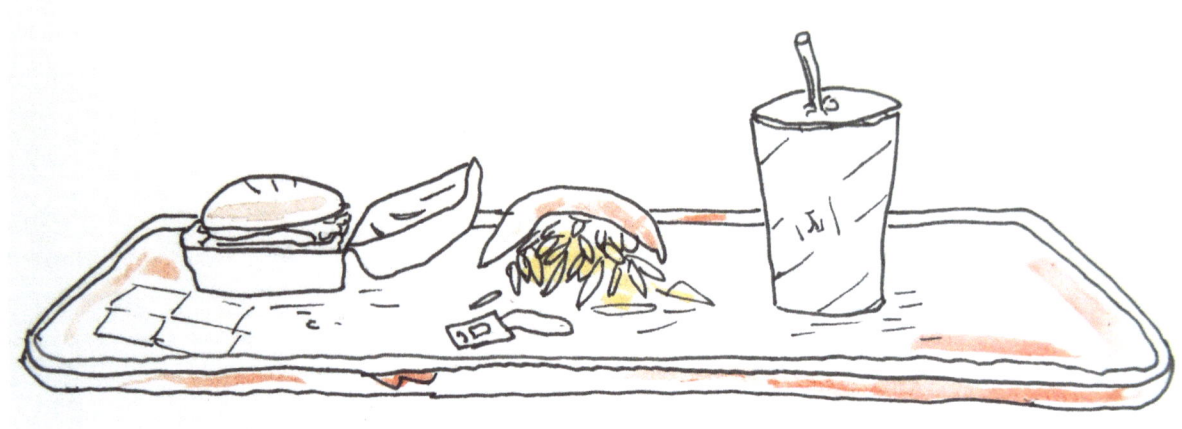

Tip 51: Let's focus on the food products. All general food advice is good for everyone, but even better for HSPs. So avoid processed and **junk food** and eat lots of **vegetables and fruits**.

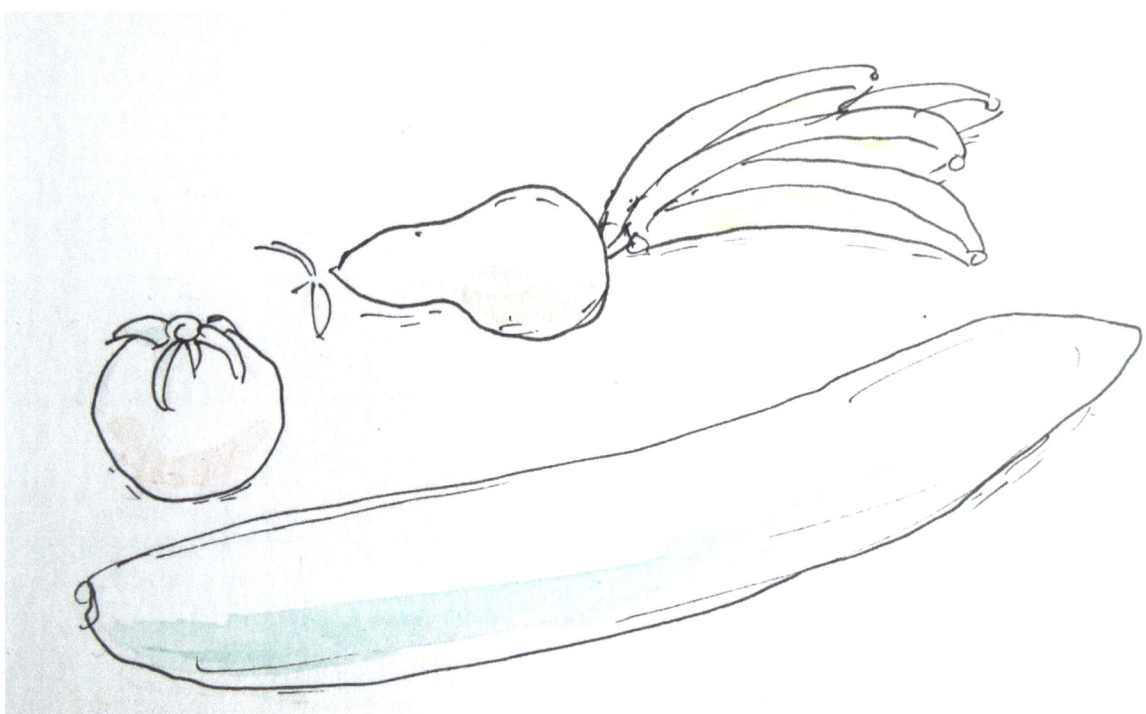

Tip 52: **Moderate**. Eating junk food every now and then isn't too bad. Just don't make it a habit.

Tip 53: Do you like sugar? Well, **artificial sugar** stimulates their eaters. As HSPs are already enough stimulation from their environment. So avoid energy bars and check the amounts of sugar on the packages of the food you're buying. You'll be surprised how much artificial sugar is present in your everyday food.

Tip 54: Fan of **chocolate**? Try to limit it, especially white and brown chocolate. Eating too much chocolate can give you difficulties sleeping.

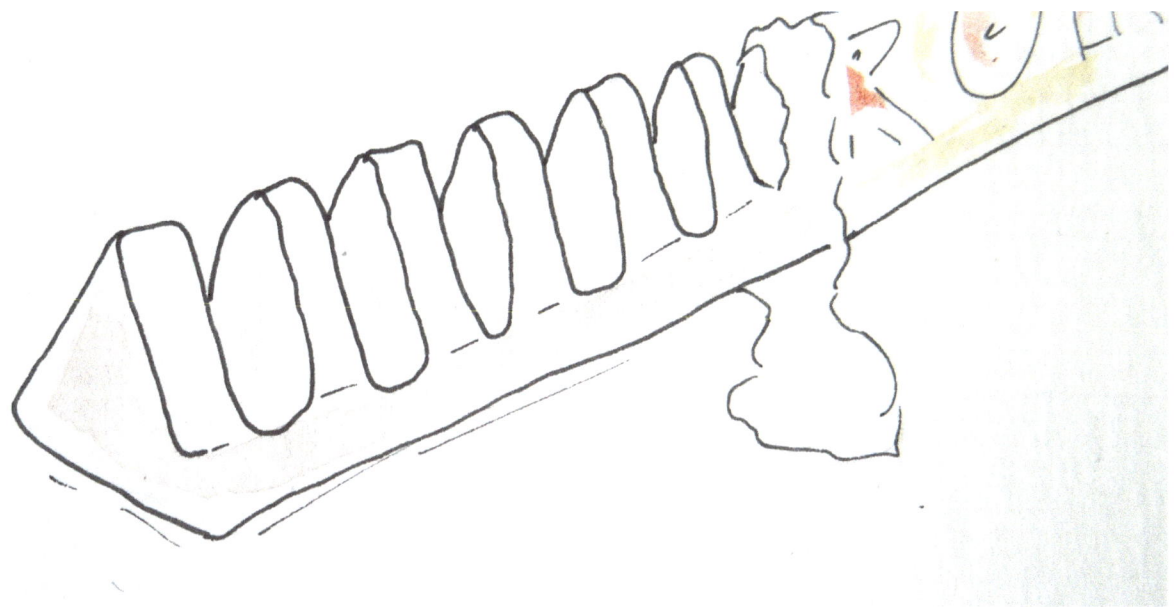

Tip 55: So what's the best kind of food to eat, even for non-HSPs? The simple answer is **organic food**. Always a good idea. More expensive, but better for the body. See if there are any providers in your neighbourhood, like an organic farm.

Tip 56: Are you checking the drinks to buy for the week? It's important to **avoid caffeine**. Caffeine, just like sugar, is like a loan. You're borrowing your future energy, making you believe it's energy you have now. But HSPs pay a higher rent on the loan than non-HSPs.

So if you really like coffee, buy decaf. And **avoid energy and soda drinks**. They contain lots of sugar and caffeine. No need to get overly stimulated. Like Coca Cola? Buy the one without sugar and caffeine. You'll notice, the package is different.

Tip 57: Alcohol works just like sugar and caffeine: it gets you overstimulated. Non-HSPs need a lot more to get excited. Better limit your intake. Or drink water in between two glasses. And choose for beers with **less alcohol**. Or even without any alcohol. Easier said than done, when group pressure is high - there's no shame in saying no.

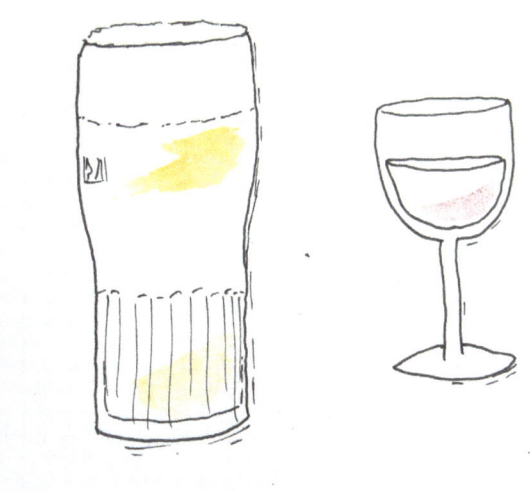

Tip 58: Since we're at the supermarket, let's go to the candles section. Buy **naturally scented candles**, to take your baths with. Or to bring a nice atmosphere to your home.

Tip 59: Last department to visit: the health and beauty section. When you're there, buy **products with organic ingredients**. Natural products are better for your body. For example, use natural fragrances (=ingredients) for deodorants and perfumes. Some HSPs can get nauseous after smelling intense, artificial perfumes.

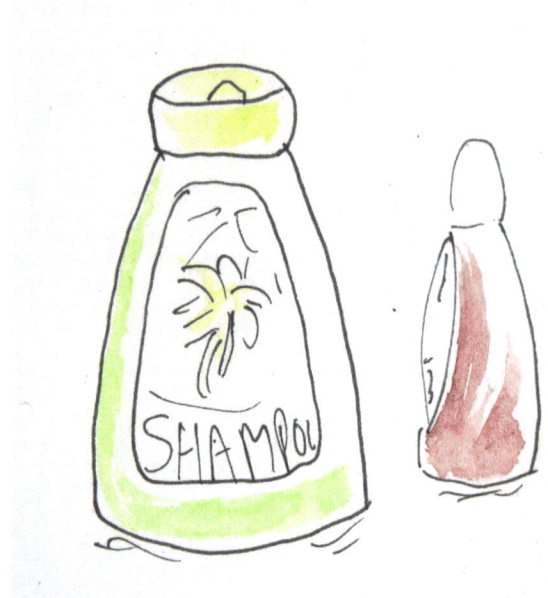

Tip 60: Put all your products in the right place in your home to avoid having visual noise. Let's see now some **hobbies**. One first tip: keep them close. The less time you commute, the better.

Tip 61: One hobby you don't need to commute much for, is **gardening**.
Spending time taking care of your garden is generally known to be a good hobby, as well for non-HSPs. Taking care of nature can be a rewarding activity. Consider having a pond. If you don't have a garden but love gardening, check if there are common gardens you can use.

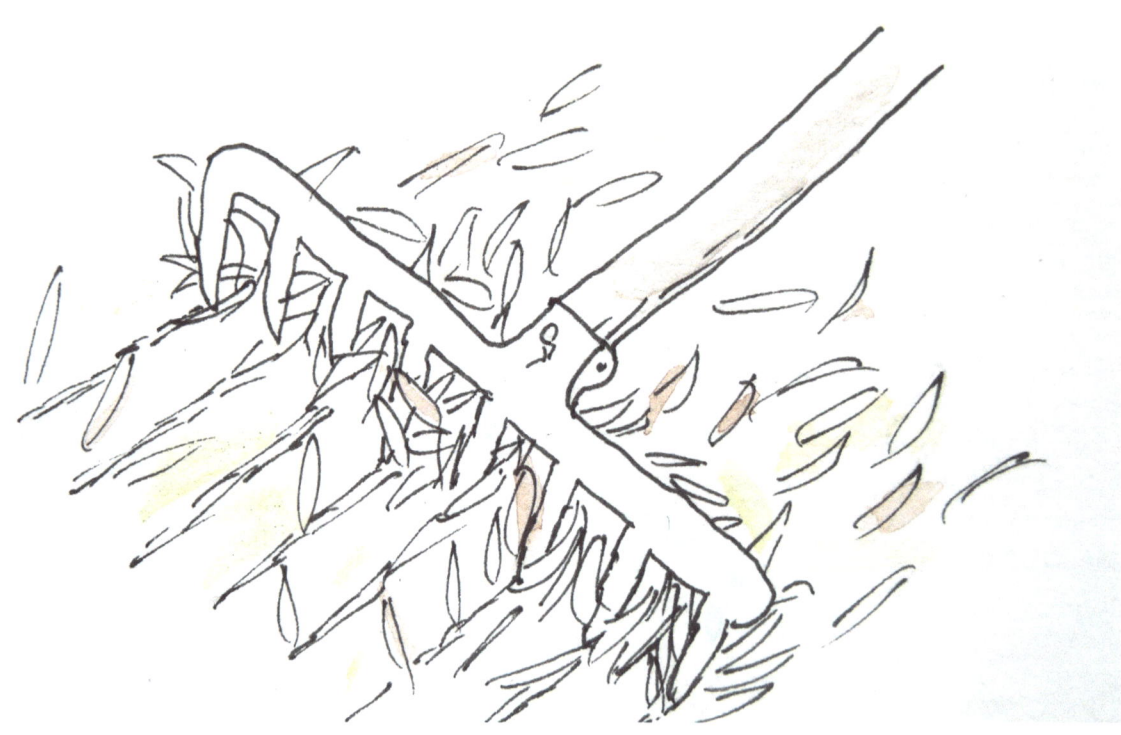

Tip 62: Love to **go out**? Some HSPs like to spend time going to nice bars, seeing people they love. If you're going out, make sure you have your own transport. So you can leave when you choose to.

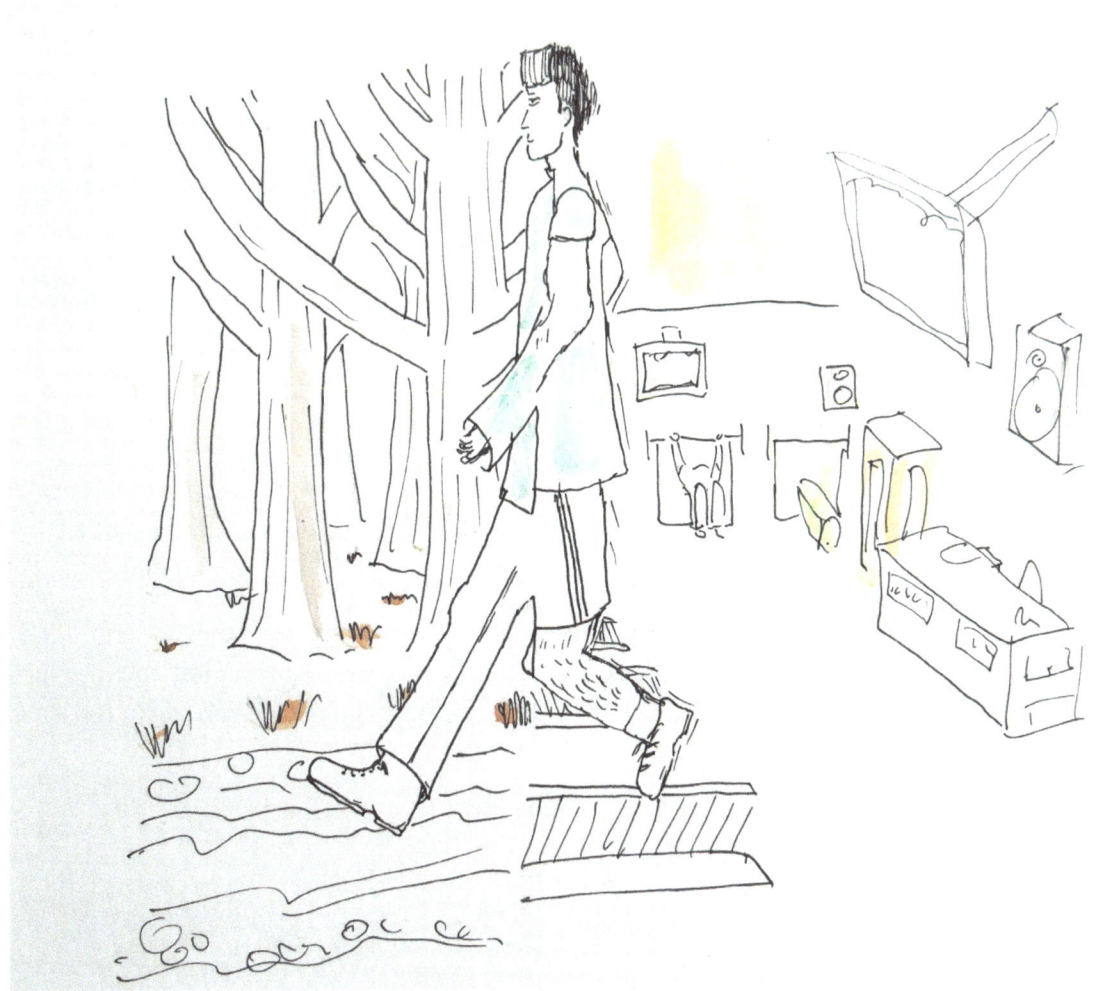

Tip 63: Hesitating between the **gym** or just a **walk**? Think about the gym for a minute. Music getting you excited. Lots of people watching. Some superficial persons. The closing hours to take into account. People exercising. And many other stimuli. To walk, you go when, where and how you please, quietness in the nature and silence. Don't forget to stretch after long walks. If you can, introduce walking into your routine.

If you like sports, mind that HSPs tend to prefer **individual sports**. Like walking, badminton or swimming. Being in a team can be great, but imagine having to pass the ball to too many other players while being challenged by the opponents, and noting the disappointment of those that didn't get the ball. Might not be your cup of tea.

So, enjoy the rest of your weekend and start your week well.

8. During the next week

Got into your weekly routine? Let's give you some food for thought to think about. At work, in the evening, or whenever it pleases you. But first, we start with a visit to the doctor.

Tip 64: Well, you don't need to go to your doctor now. Have you already checked your **allergies**? The next visit to your family doctor might be an opportunity. It will allow you to discover which ingredients you're not supposed to eat. Also tell your doctor you're an HSP.

Tip 65: Whenever your doctor prescribes medication, and you feel something unusual, check the **side-effects** of the medication. It will comfort you if you need to go more often to the bathroom, or if you're dizzy.

Tip 66: No need to consult the doctor for the use of **drugs**. Simple. Just don't. You're more sensitive to them than non-HSPs. And they're not healthy anyway.

Let's give yourself some time to reflect on **a few ideas** that can improve your life as an HSP. They will take quite a while to have a good result, so don't expect results immediately.

Tip 67: Where do you go when you're overwhelmed? When you have bad news, or an argument that didn't go as planned, or another conflict, **where's your spot**? Find one in your home. Not necessarily a whole room. Put some personal belongings there. And make it a habit of going there when you need to.

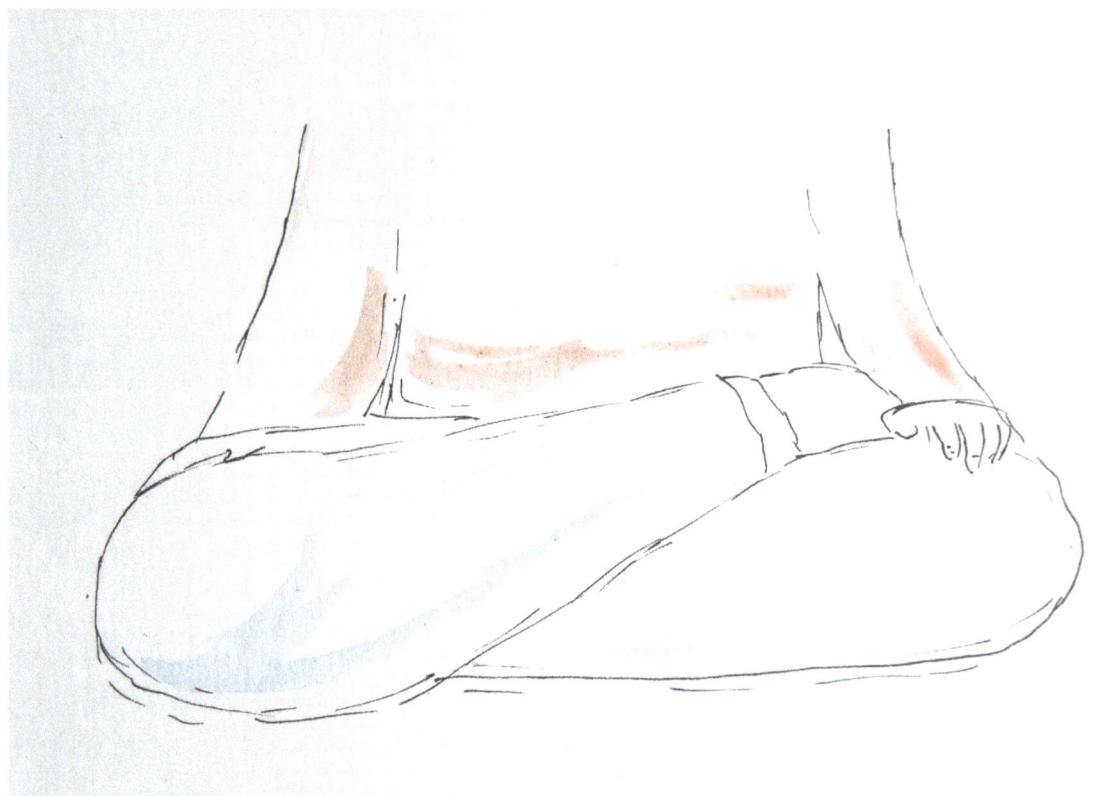

Tip 68: How do you calm down? In today's world, there are many ways to find **relaxation**. Yoga, mindfulness and meditation are just some of them. Try different options to find the one you feel best with. That lets you reconnect with your body. Make it part of your routine - morning or evening, what fits best for you.

One aspect about relaxation that is very important, is **breathing** well. It has many advantages, for example you'll feel less stressed. Many persons breathe through their chest. But it's much better to breathe through the belly. Find breathing techniques on the internet. You can start by searching for stomach or abdominal breathing. Also do them while working. Again, this is a long-term investment - so make them part of your routine.

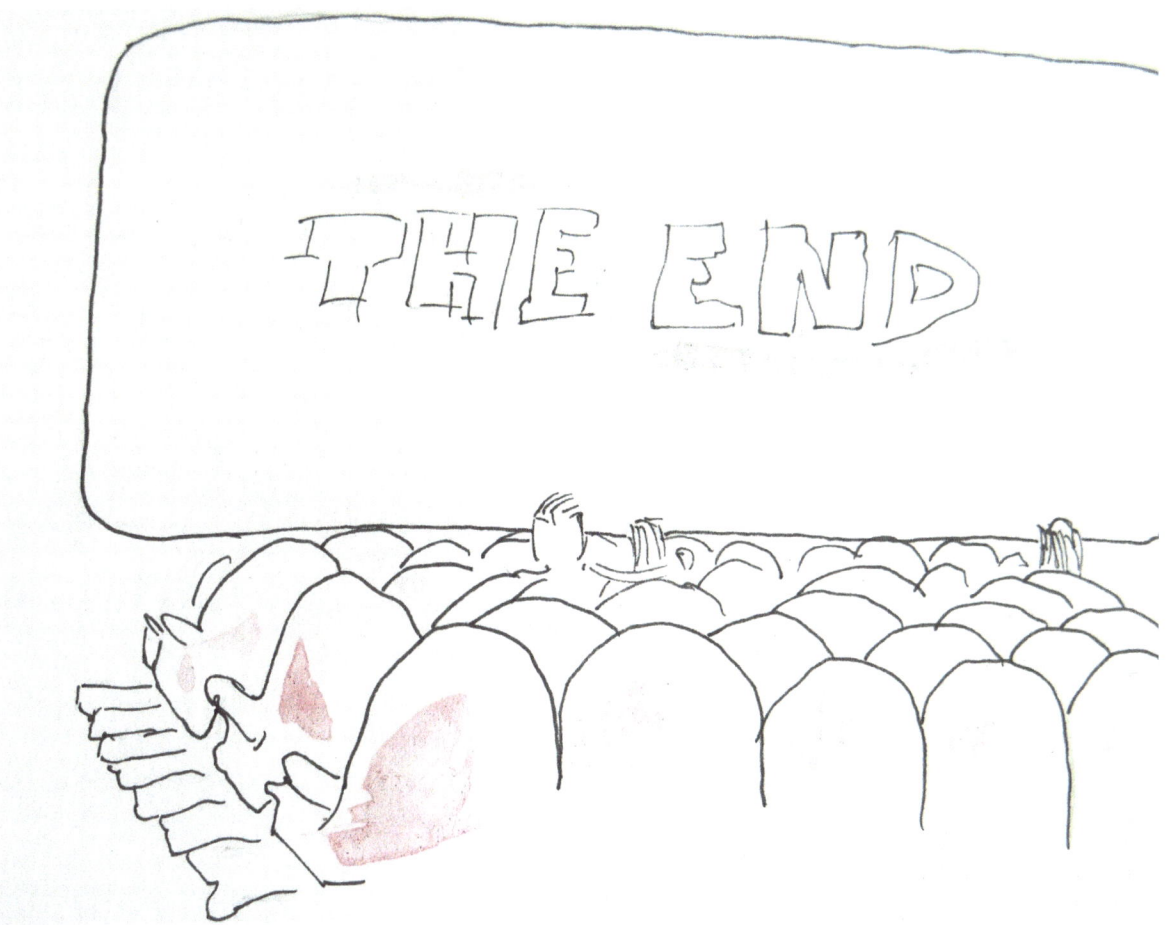

Tip 69: Like to go to the **movies**? Check out which days are more quiet. And go in the room just when the film starts. No need to see those commercials. And hear the eating noises of others.

Tip 70: Love good air? Spend time in your **garden**. It's not only because of the fresh air. Noises don't echo. Nature is around. So it's a great place for an HSP. Maybe you could do your relaxation outside. If you don't have a garden, check if there's a park in your neighbourhood.

Tip 71: While you're in the garden, think if you can **grow your own food**. It's good for many reasons. You'll develop a better routine, you'll feel fulfilment as you're taking care of nature, and the food is generally better. Which will give you additional satisfaction. Also think of growing your own spices.

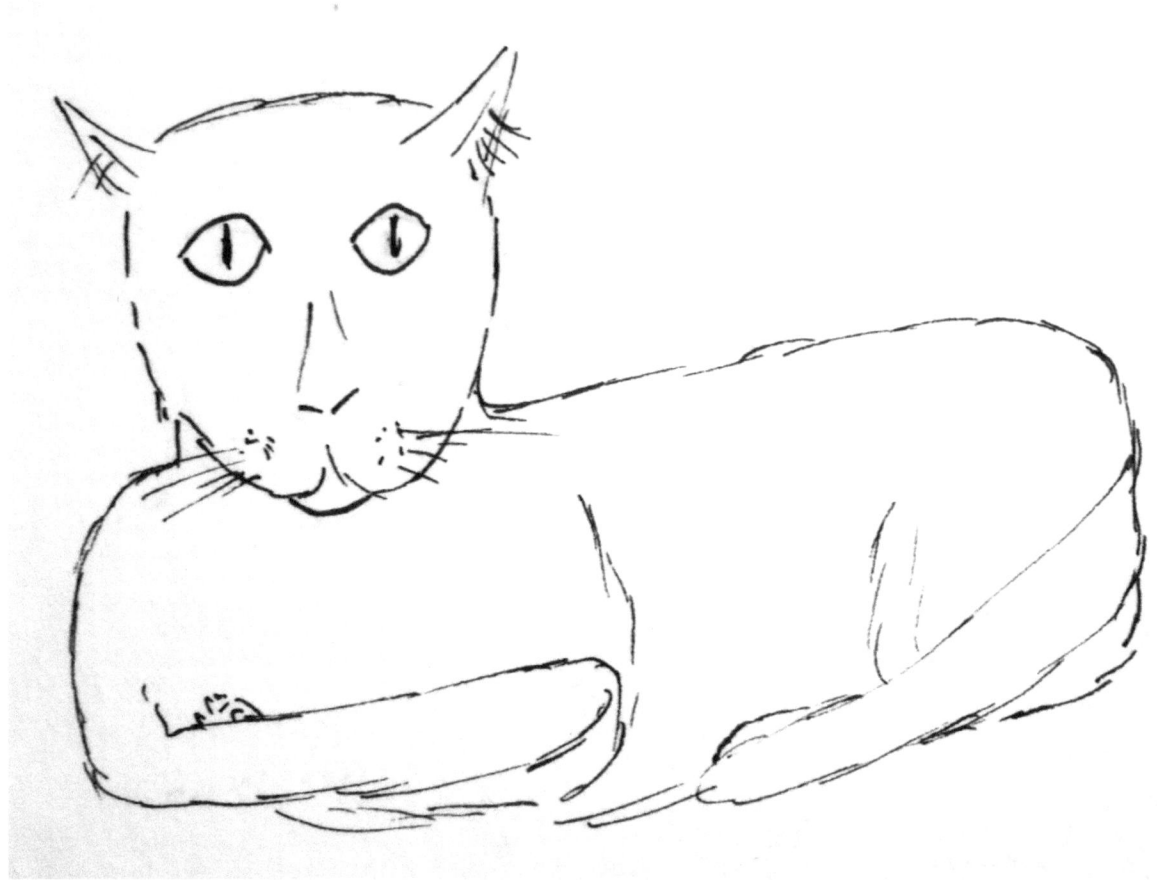

Tip 72: Last tip for this week to think about: consider **having a pet**. Pets are like plants. They don't judge but need to be taken care of. Something HSPs love to do. They can give compassion when you're a little down. One tip though: don't buy or adopt a barking dog. Also: cats fight and scream when they mate. So adopt one according to your preferences.

So here's your to do-list for this week. Well, it's more a to-think-list:

- Do I have an own spot in my house? How do I feel there?

- What relaxation methods have I already tried? Which one was best? Which one could I try (again)?

- Which breathing technique would I start trying?

- Which vegetables, fruits and spices could I grow? Which do I want to grow?

- Which pet would I want? What are the pro's and con's?

9. The weekend after

After all the thinking, a well-deserved weekend. To go shopping! Last weekend, we went to the supermarket. This weekend, it's time to go to hardware and decoration stores. Don't hesitate to go to specialised stores. Afterwards, we'll pay a visit to a music store. But first, find stores where you can find the following items for your home.

Tip 73: Buy **white drapes and curtains**. You can hang white drapes on the windows which can be seen by strangers, so you'll have your privacy. When it's dark, close the curtains. Buy curtains that absorb sound and light, so a full moon won't keep you awake. And avoid blinds, as they make unnecessary sound, for example when there's wind.

Tip 74: Buy **mosquito screens**. Mosquitoes horribly disturb many HSPs' sleep. An anti-insect screen on your window and closed doors can prevent it. Better and more natural than a chemical spray. If not at home, remember they look for warmth to get through the night. So they'll look for warm bricks when temperatures fall in the evening. Close your door then.

Maybe you haven't thought of it before. But as an HSP, the nicer you make your home, the nicer it will be for the persons you're living with. Or visitors. So you're doing it in the first place for yourself, but others will benefit too.

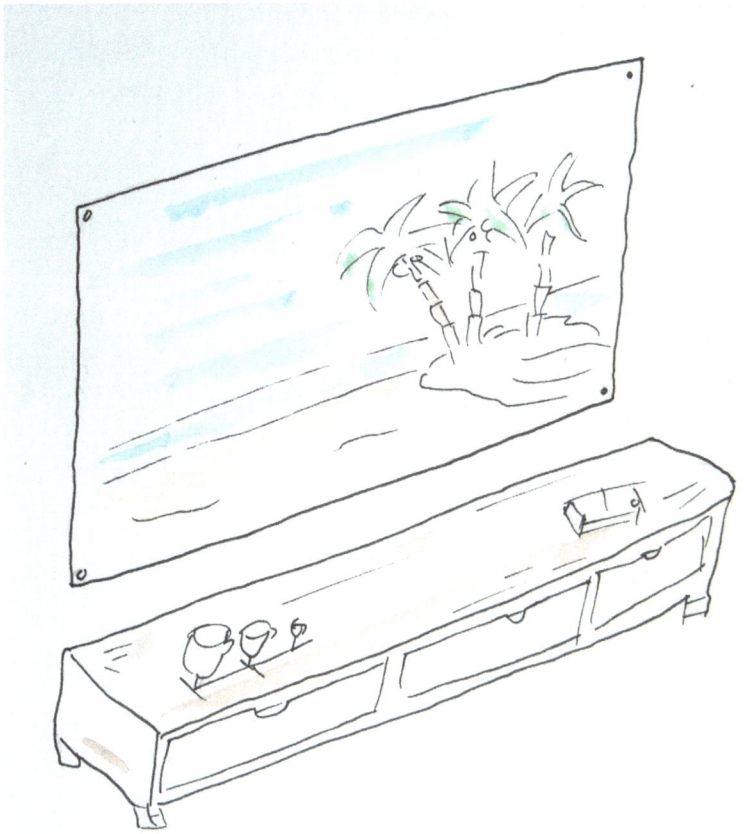

Tip 75: Buy nice **posters**. Hang big posters or paintings around your house. Preferably those that show natural beauty. For example: a waterfall, a view of snowy mountains, a Mediterranean sunset or the Amazon forest. These views can have a calming effect. Don't hang too many though. And make sure to do this at work as well.

Tip 76: Have you thought of what **colours the walls** have in your home? Colours can affect your mood as well as your stress levels. Fluorescent colours as well as red, orange and yellow can provoke unnecessary emotions. So better avoid them. Search on the internet for calming or soothing colours before buying paint. Also mind that changing rooms can lead to a loss of energy for HSPs. So aim at colours that are in harmony with each other.

Tip 77: Buy **rugs**. Choose those with nice patterns and colours that fit in the room they're lying in. Rugs absorb noise - which is something HSPs want to reduce as much as possible. Moreover, sound, unlike light, doesn't stop when it meets a wall.

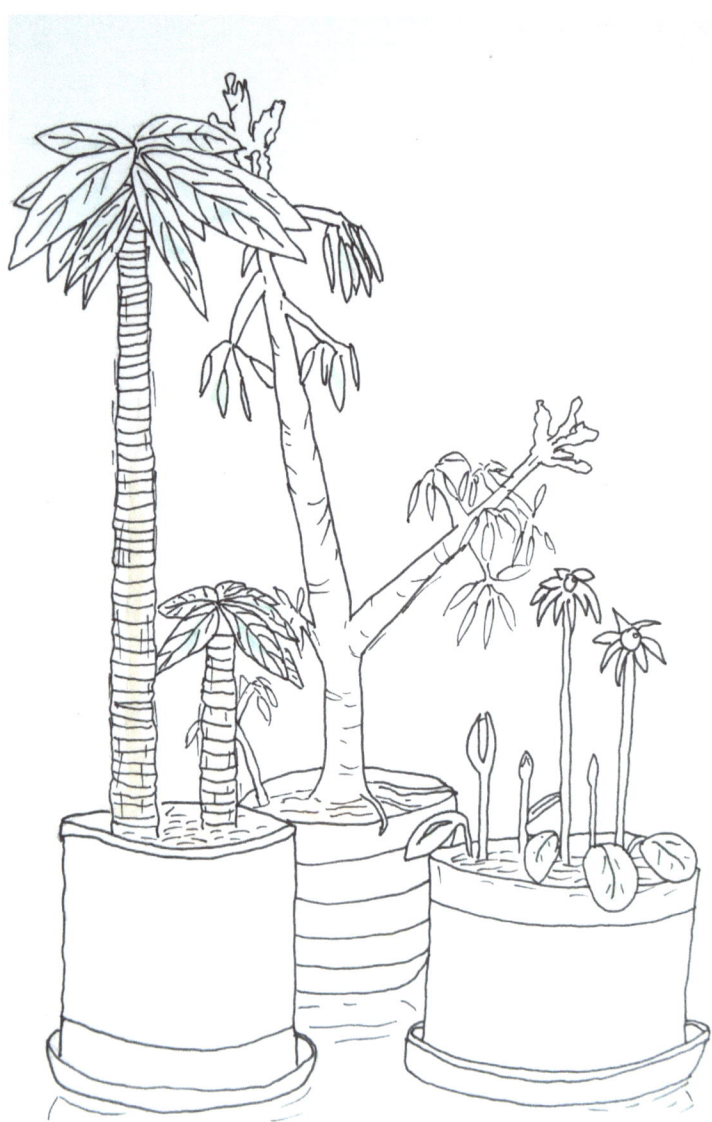

Tip 78: Put plants everywhere. **Plants** are made for HSPs. They clean the air. They calm your mood. They never judge anyone. They embellish your home. They need to be taken care of. They give you routine. But avoid fake plants. And don't exaggerate. You might lose track of who needs water when.

Tip 79: Do you hear a lot of noise from your **pillow** when you're trying to sleep? Certain pillows just make noise. If so, buy new ones, lay your head on them and move a bit. Noisy? Try another one until you find the right one. This will avoid you to have sleepless nights.

Tip 80: We're almost out of the hardware and decoration stores. One last item to buy: **taps** that don't drip. The sound of drips can get HSPs off. So either learn how to repair your tap, or buy a tap that doesn't drip. Or something to catch the drip without sound.

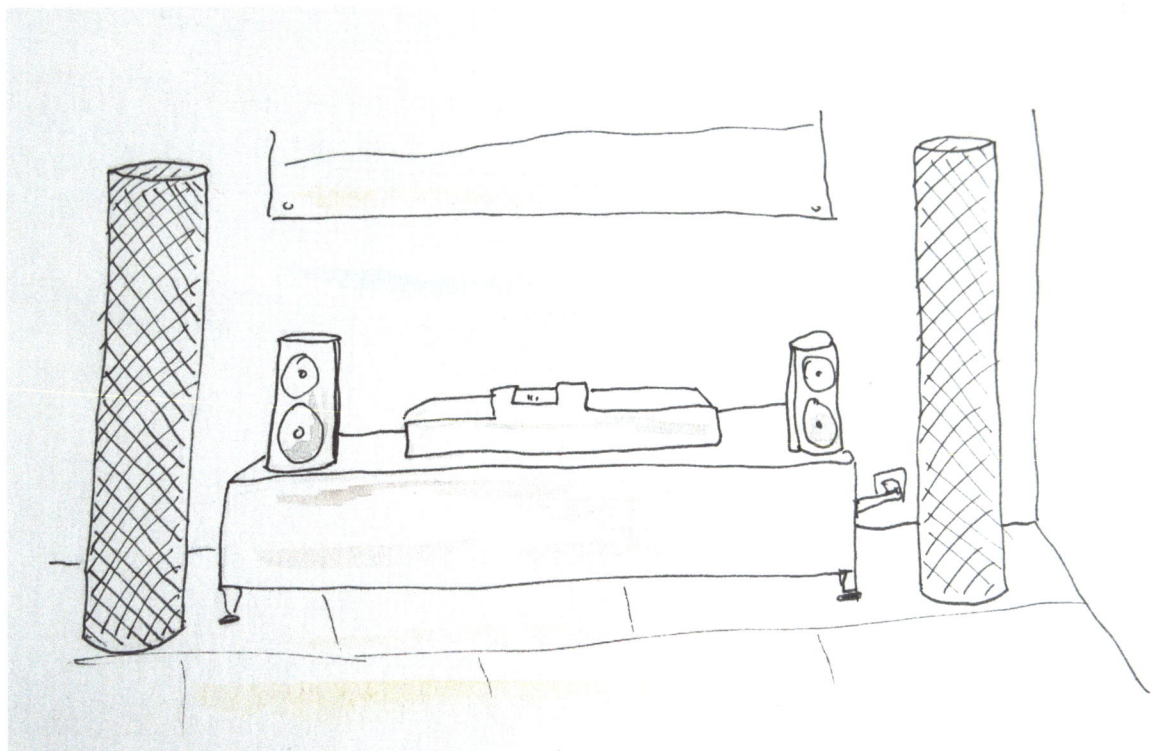

Tip 81: Next stop: the music shop. When you feel those chills listening to your favourite music, that's typically something for HSPs. For non-HSPs, it's really hard to get them. So enjoy it. Buy a **stereo** with loudspeakers as big as you like.

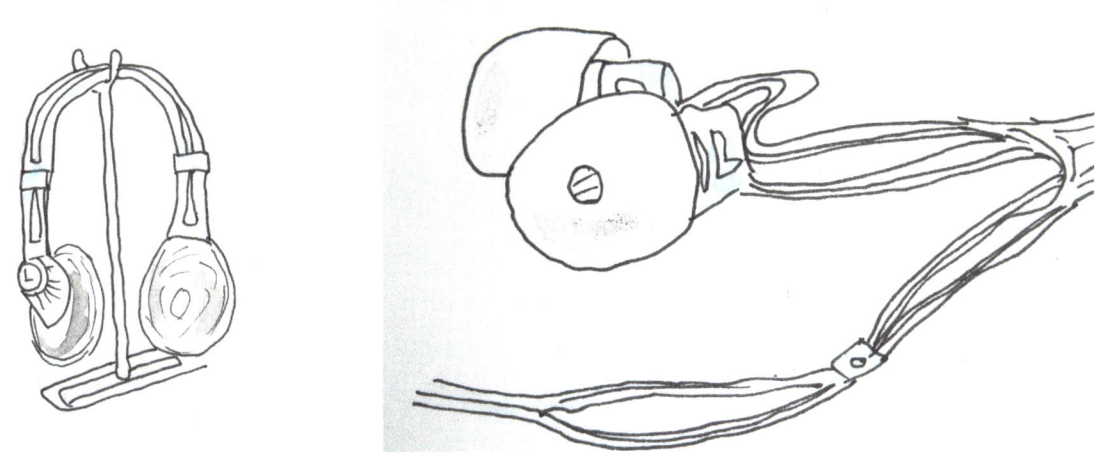

Tip 82: Buy high-quality **headphones** and noise-reducing **earplugs**. Headphones are very handy if your neighbours are too close and have a different taste. Earplugs reduce the amount of noise. If necessary, go to a specialised shop to have them custom-made so they will filter out particular types of noise.

Well, that's enough work for the weekend.

10. The second week after

The weekend is over, so it's time to think again how you can improve your home to make it more yours. Let's see some other ideas that will require you to think about how you want to live.

Tip 83: How can you use your **creative skills** to embellish your home? HSPs tend to have a lot of imagination. If you like to paint, hang those you choose on the wall. If you like to take pictures, print and hang them around your home. If you don't want to shop them, that's ok too. Many artists are HSPs. So why not do it yourself, as a hobby, in the comfort of your own home, where no one is watching? It's also a good way to express your emotions.

Tip 84: One way of expression is by **playing music**. Choose electric music instruments. Playing electric instruments not only reduce the sound, but you can also make sure no one is listening to you while you're learning to play.

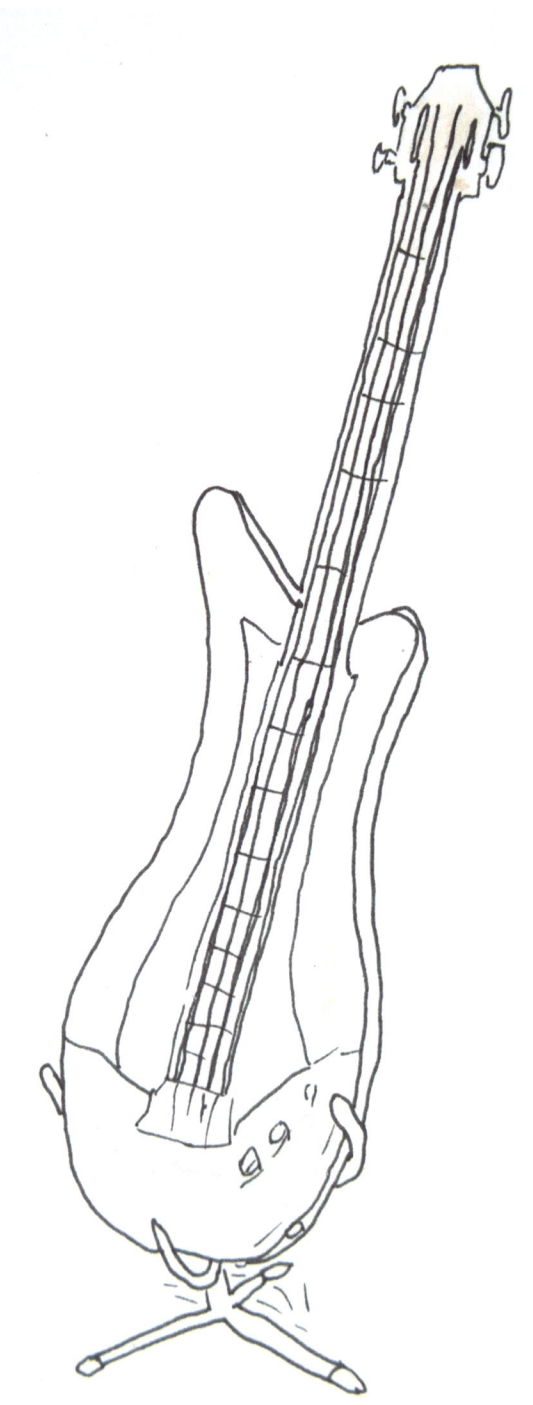

Tip 85: Apart from being creative, **decorate** your home. Use objects you like to touch. Or those that have a positive meaning to you. Or to watch. Or those that absorb sound. A library with many interesting books is an example.

Tip 86: Do you have big rooms with bare walls and hard floors? Those rooms might have an **echo**. All sounds replicate themselves because they're not absorbed. When you're decorating, mind this. Put large objects to break the sound. Or even acoustic foam panels. Also, big, empty rooms allow many persons to come together. Which is something some HSPs can't stand.

Tip 87: Do you have a place to show your **collections**, like your books? HSPs love to collect. So make sure there's space for your collections.

Let's see how **work and home** are related. Work makes many HSPs feel uncomfortable. Understandable, since colleagues make noise. They do office politics. They talk about each other. And worst of all: you can hear it all. At home, none of these problems happen.

Tip 88: So you could consider **working from home**. For HSPs, it's a privilege to be able to work from home. No colleagues watching you. No commute so no annoying traffic jams. No open office workspaces. Even if it's only for one day a week, for example by teleworking, it can already be a relief.

Tip 89: Even better than working from home is to **work at home**. Meaning, your job is at home. Many professions can be done at home. Like translators. Or therapists. You can combine it with a part-time job outside of your home. Make sure the place where you work is nicely decorated.

Tip 90: If you can't work at home, it's important to have a job **close to where you live**. Commuting is usually not a good thing for HSPs, especially long commutes. Because there's the lack of control - will the bus be there on time? Will there be a lot of people on the train?

Tip 91: What do you prefer: a **smart** or a **classic phone**? Smart has access to the internet, takes decent pictures and has many applications. However, batteries don't last, they're expensive, only last 1-2 years and break easily. With classic phones, no hacking, no wifi needed, no work emails, less endless conversations and more 'real' conversations, especially when you're going out. So choose the one that's the most convenient for you.

So now ask yourself the following questions this week:

• What creative hobby do I like? Drawing? Writing? Painting? How can I use those for my home?

• Which instrument do I want to play? Which songs or pieces do I want to play?

• What's my preferred decoration store? What do I like about the decoration that's there? Is there enough room for it in my home?

• What part of my work can I do at home? When can I ask my boss to work more from home? Can I work part-time? What job do I really like? Which job could I do part-time from home?

• Why do I really need a smartphone? What would I lose if I used a classic phone?

11. The weeks after

Let's see some other practical tips to use at the right time - not necessarily this week or the next. A first example is the time of the year.

Tip 92: Different **seasons** have different consequences. Snow means you can enjoy the silence. During spring, many smells come to you. And enjoy the colours of autumn leaves. However, adapt your behaviour. Walk slower when it's hot. And take a walk during winter. When it's warm enough, **eat in the garden**. It's usually a more peaceful spot than inside.

Tip 93: When **seasons change**, HSPs can be extra vulnerable. Same goes for sudden temperature changes. Make sure to take extra vitamins in the beginning of the winter.

Tip 94: Seasons changing can be an opportunity to **decorate** again. Have fun decorating a Christmas tree in December.

Tip 95: Like to **travel**? Make sure to rest enough. Your routine is disrupted. You'll see other places, giving extra stimuli. Jet lags are more difficult to process for HSPs. So make sure to prepare for your travels. Scheduling a day of rest during and after your travel isn't a bad idea. Especially if you travel far away.

If you take a plane, take a **window seat**. Less people passing by just next to you. A window to gaze at. And you can put your head against the wall to rest.

Tip 96: **Fashion or not to fashion**? Interesting question. Finding the right clothes can be very rewarding. Many HSPs work in fashion thanks to their fine taste and their ability to spot new trends. Others hate shopping: the music and constantly changing environments don't help.

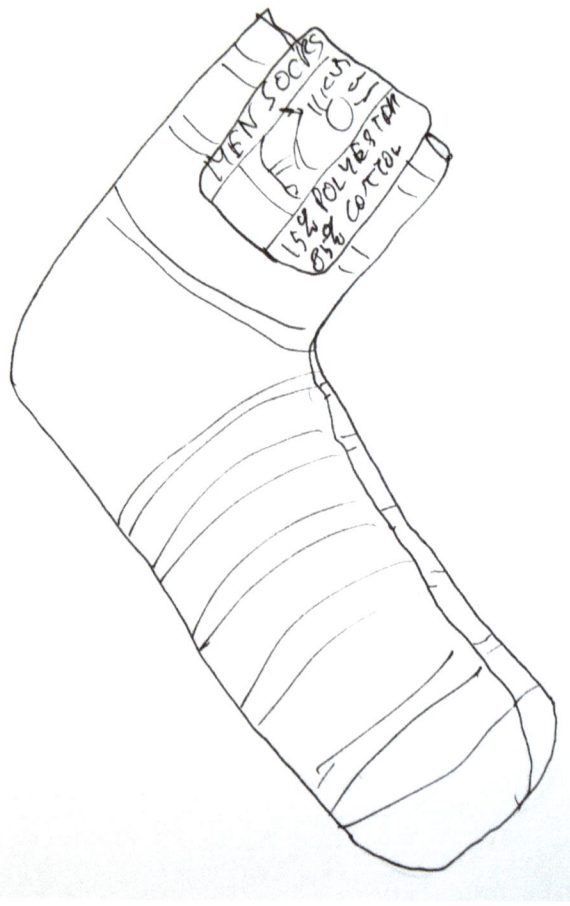

Tip 97: When you're buying clothes, make sure to avoid substances that make you uncomfortable, especially **polyester**. It can make HSPs sweat excessively.

Tip 98: Choose your **shopping hours** wisely. And try to go when you don't really need new clothes, it will keep the pressure off.

Tip 99: As soon as you have bought clothes, make sure to **remove the labels** if they bug you. Some HSPs can get upset by those labels.

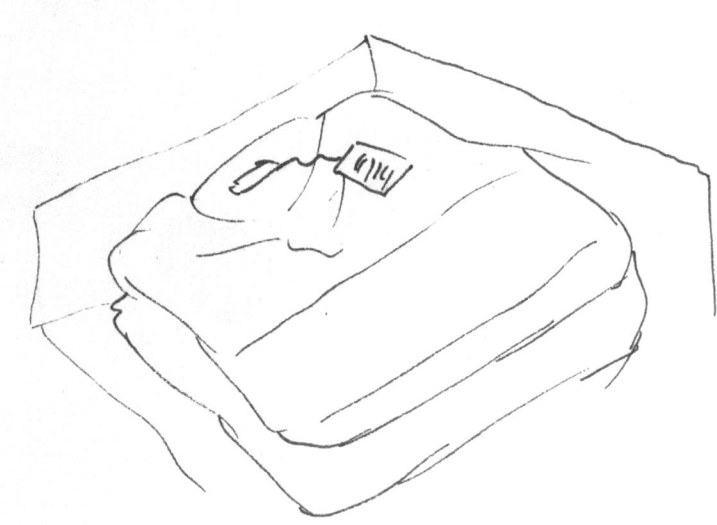

Tip 100: How do you like your **haircuts**? Avoid busy hours and ask for a quiet spot near natural light. So you won't be as much affected by the many clients, the loud music and the noises everywhere multiplied by the number of mirrors. Another idea is to look for a hairdresser that comes to your home. Or a private hairdresser.

Some questions to ask yourself about these last tips:

- What effect do the seasons have on me? Do I adapt enough? What do I enjoy about the different seasons?

- What kind of vacations do I love to take? Staying at home? Or going far away? Do I take enough rest while on vacation?

- Do I enjoy the clothes I usually buy? Am I sensitive to certain materials? How do I feel after shopping? Which shops did I enjoy the most?

So that's the last of the 100 tips! Let's go to the bonus sections for more inspiration…

Bonus 1: Choose your home wisely

Everyone wants to get a nice house for a low price. However, for HSPs, it's not just buying or renting and signing a contract. Or putting a few bricks together. When you're searching for a home, mind the following advice.

Tip 1: The **environment** matters. Near a busy or a crowded road? Trains and trams passing every day? Sirens from the hospital or the police station? Many houses under construction? Motorbike club in the neighbourhood? All bad signs. Try to find a home near nature. A lake, a river, a quiet playground or even a fountain can bring peace in your everyday life.

Tip 2: Before building, buying or renting, **talk to the neighbours**. They'll be able to tell you how the neighbourhood is. If you're living in an apartment, you may want to avoid living under persons walking around in high heels or who like to play their music loudly and organise weekly parties. Even a dishwasher can get an HSP angry.

So good relations with neighbours can always come handy. So that you're not blocked between your anger and your tendency to avoid conflict. Also pass a few times at different times of the day to hear the **noise levels**.

Tip 3: If you're planning to **share** an apartment, it's very important to feel comfortable with the people you're living with. So ask them questions about the things you care about before renting.

Tip 4: Looking for a home in the **city or** in a **small town**? In the city, there are more activities. But you will find more quietness in a small town. Where you might be more subject to gossip. Try to find a place according to your needs.

Tip 5: Check if the house has **double-glazed windows**. Definitely better than single-glazed windows. These windows will keep the heat in during winter and out during summer. Keeping a constant temperature is best for HSPs.

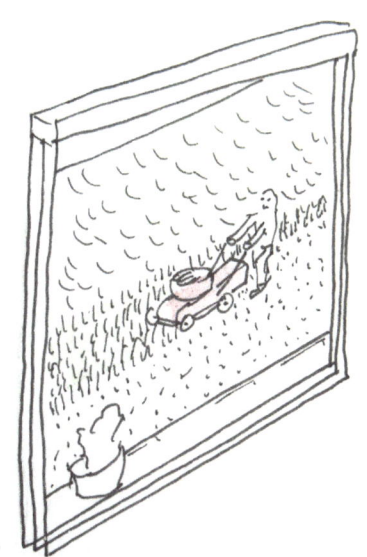

Triple-glazed windows are more expensive, but just that bit better than double-glazed. Especially for keeping the noise out. However, make sure that your walls are enough isolated. No point in upgrading to triple-glazed if it's easier for the cold to come in via the walls anyway.

Tip 6: Choose a radiator or air-conditioning that doesn't make **irritating noises**. Same for those small, portable heaters. Consider wearing an extra pull-over instead.

Tip 7: Choose a home with **windows** that are big enough. To let lots of natural light in.

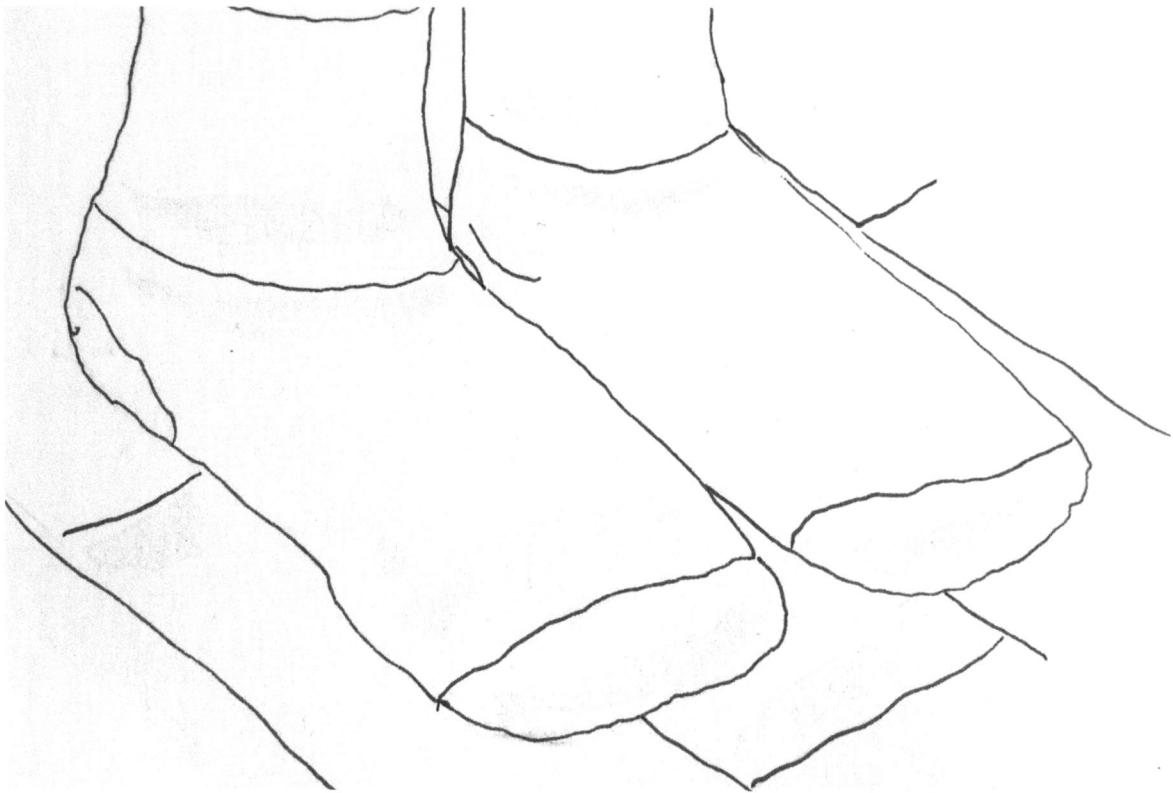

Tip 8: Cold feet can give you a cold. So don't forget to wear socks. Or if you can, invest in **floor heating**.

Questions about your home to reflect upon:

- Which neighbourhoods would I love to live in? Do I like where I live? How are my neighbours?

- What should I pay attention when looking for a new place to live? How can I prepare for it? What would be the most important requirements to write on my checklist? How can I check the neighbourhood first?

- What 'big changes' did I always want to make to my house? How much would they cost? Will they really improve the way I live?

Bonus 2: Kids in the house

Many HSPs have a love-hate relationships with children. On the one hand, they don't judge the HSPs and are easy to connect with. Children haven't got used to small talk, which HSPs usually don't like too much. On the other hand, crying babies, smelly diapers, kids running in all directions are stimuli HSPs have difficulties processing. The lack of control also plays its part. However, HSPs tend to be great parents. For example, it's easier to 'tune' in the needs of the children. So let's see some tips for kids.

Tip 1: Don't forget to **work on yourself**. Children mirror their parents. That's why your first task is to take care of yourself, for example with the relevant tips in this book. So if you don't accept yourself, your children will also have difficulties accepting themselves. Focus on being a good parent, not on directly satisfying all your children's needs.

Tip 2: When you need to have some time on your own, **explain me-time**. The better they understand you need time for yourself, the better they will understand they need time alone themselves too. Same goes for respect. The earlier you teach them this, the better.

Tip 3: Do you have a **baby** that **cries** too much? Babies can be held in a particular position, which resembles to the baby's position in the womb. Hold them like that to make them stop crying. Tick in 'quiet baby position' in Google to find more information and videos.

Tip 4: Don't buy **too many books**. HSPs tend to buy to many books to educate their children. Sometimes, the advices contradict one another. This will confuse you. And there's no need for that.

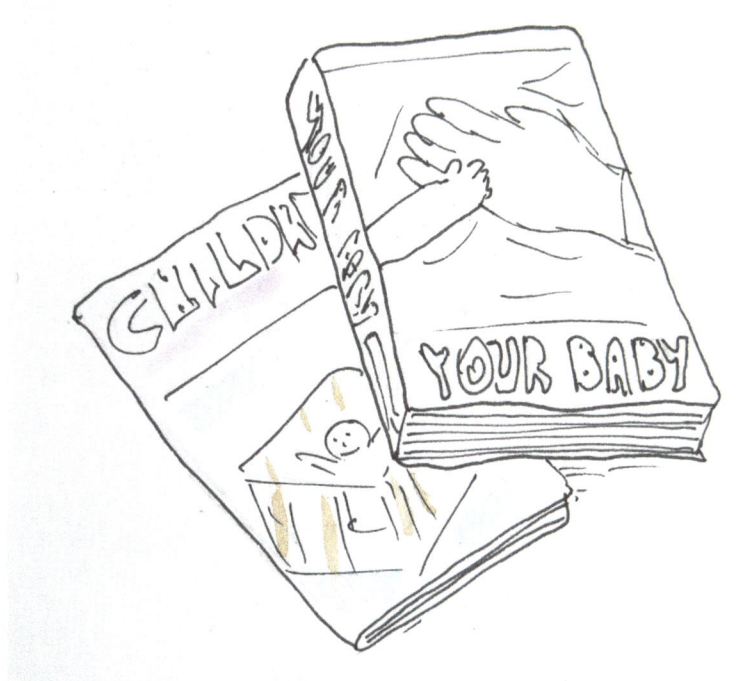

Tip 5: Check when the you're the **busiest** with your children. Usually the morning rush and just before dinner. Prepare and think how you can cope better. For example, by letting your children play the same game just before eating. Or having your earplugs ready.

Tip 6: Let your children use their energy **in the garden** as much as possible. Or in the park. Inside, it's easier to get tense.

Tip 7: Make sure to **limit the access to their toys**. Only allow them access to a part of the toys. It limits the visual noise and makes it easier to tidy up. Also determine limits on where they can play.

Tip 8: Regularly start bigger activities with **one rule or limit**. For example, no playing in the kitchen. Or: no feet in the couch. Or: only one hour watching TV. The idea is that you establish your authority, which may be challenging for HSPs.

If the kids don't respect the rule, make sure to discipline them. You will normally only have to do it once. Afterwards, the kids will know you stick by your rules and they will accept your authority. It will make parenting much easier.

Tip 9: Say **no to noise-toys**. Children can also play with those that don't make any noise. Don't buy batteries for the toys - they make noise.

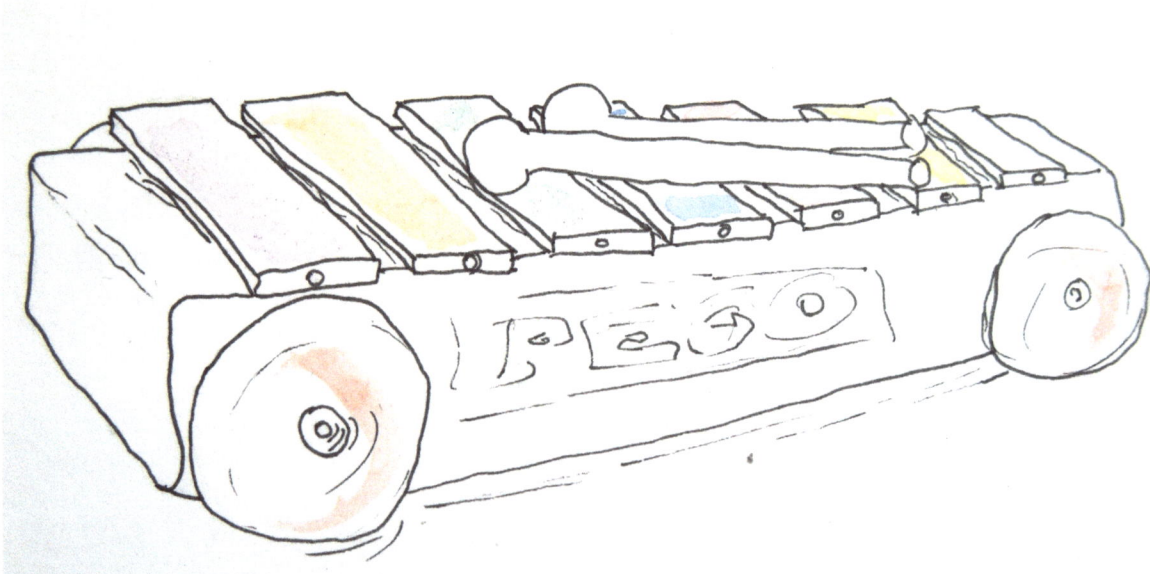

Tip 10: **Involve your kids** with activities they might like around the house. If you suspect they might be HSP, involve them in activities like painting or cooking. If they're not, make sure to let them do activities they like. But don't forget your limits.

Tip 11: Before sleeping, let them find and talk about **one thing they did well** during the day. They'll sleep better. You can do the same for yourself.

Reflect about the following questions about your kids:

• Do they accept that I need time on my own? Can you talk about this with them? Do they respect you for who you are? Do you have enough time for yourself? How can you increase that time if you need to?

• Can you show your emotions in the right way to your children?

• How do you enjoy your time with your children? How can you increase this? Which activities you enjoy can you share with your children?

To finish: don't forget to use all the other tips of the book. For example, earplugs can be lifesavers. But it's so easy to forget about them while you have kids crying.

Bonus 3: interesting links

Elaine Aron, one of the leading scientists conducting HSP research, has a website with tests to check your level of sensitivity:

- hsperson.com

- hsperson.com/test

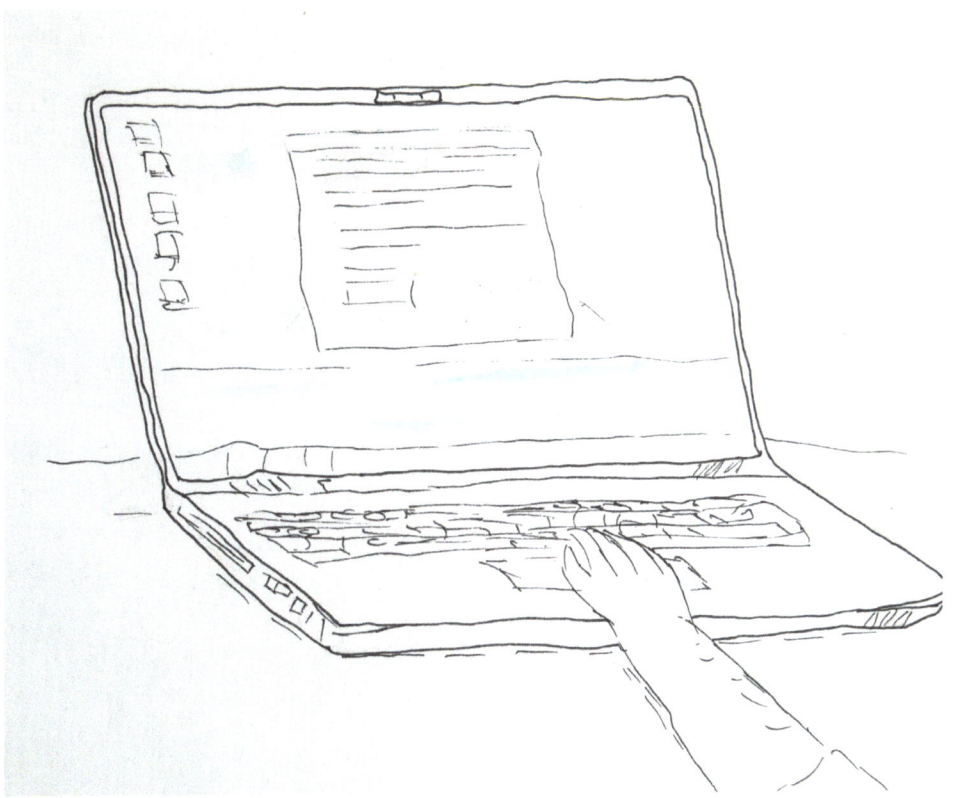

Many tips, podcasts and more on:

- highlysensitivepeople.com

- highlysensitiveperson.net

- highlysensitive.org

- An interesting website with many other links.

And here are my links:

- My website with additional tips, advice and inspiration.

- My YouTube channel: inspirational videos and advice.

- My online course: a course covering different aspects of being and living as an HSP.

- My books: a collection of my books.

The final word - About the author

We're at the end of the book, hope you have found and applied some tips that make your life as a very sensitive person easier.

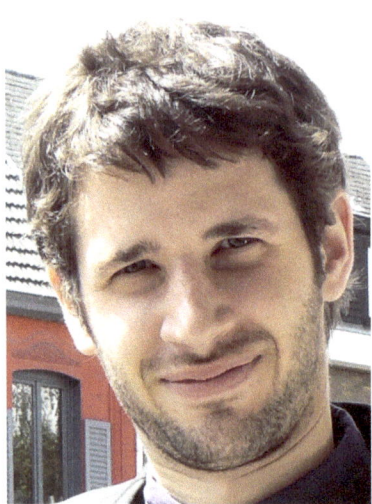

Alain de Raymond discovered his sensitivity when he borrowed one of Elaine Aron's books at the local library by accident. It gave him the inspiration to share his tips in this book, as well as on a video channel and in an online course. His aim is to let people discover themselves and to help them grow as individuals.

He loves learning languages, drawing, music and many other fine arts. He drew the images in this book.

Except being sensitive, he loves economics, politics and all the processes that shape society. He worked in communications a few years and holds 3 degrees: in Journalism, EU Studies and Management.

Cover picture (https://pixabay.com/en/woman-girl-bella-read-sleep-2197947/) and in the introduction are in the public domain. Drawings & picture above © Alain de Raymond.